High Praise for
Sometimes My Heart Goes Numb

"Danny, Eric, Micaela, Bharat—I wanted to meet each of these exemplary caregivers and say, 'thank you' for demonstrating that we have an astonishing capacity for love. Here are twenty people who, in the face of life's greatest challenges, show us what to do, what to say, and how to be a compassionate presence when there is little that can be said or done. *Sometimes My Heart Goes Numb* is one of the most practical, well-written and moving books I've ever read."

—Paula Van Ness, president, the National AIDS Fund,
  Washington, D.C.

"*Sometimes My Heart Goes Numb* is the finest book yet written on the human side of caring for people with life-threatening illnesses. It offers riveting and informative stories about loved ones, friends, health professionals and community volunteers at their compassionate best. Charles Garfield picks up where *And the Band Played On* left off and transports us beyond the mind-numbing numbers and often callous rhetoric straight to the heart of one of the most compelling challenges of our generation. This book is a must-read for those living with HIV/AIDS, those caring for someone infected and, most certainly, those who believe that offering love and service to men, women, and children in need is still a part of the American dream."

—Bill Freeman, executive director,
  National Association of People with AIDS, Washington, D.C.

"*Sometimes My Heart Goes Numb* talks straight from the heart with compassion, wisdom, and courage. If someone you love has AIDS, this is *the* book to read."

—Dushan Angius, chair, Rotary AIDS Project

"People everywhere owe a debt of gratitude to AIDS caregivers be they nurses, friends, lovers, or neighbors. Everyone who cares for someone with AIDS will be uplifted by this extraordinary book."

—Don Francis, M.D., D.Sc., Genentech, Inc.,
   retired from the Centers for Disease Control

"An extremely valuable source of information for all of us. If you are alive, you are a caregiver. Read on; laugh, cry, grow, and learn how to deal with life's afflictions. Your heart will be touched and your mind opened. When you read the stories contained in this book, you will become passionate about life, not numb."

—Bernie Siegel, M.D., author of *Love, Medicine, and Miracles*

"Here's a collection of stories about extraordinary heroes facing what is rapidly becoming America's most ordinary cause of death. It is a tribute to them that while others took refuge in fear and judgmentalism, they took action with courage and skill. And it is a tribute to Garfield that after all the suffering and dying he has witnessed, he still calls to comfort me when I feel alone . . . he has never allowed his heart to go numb."

—Mary Fisher, founder, The Family AIDS Network,
   author of *Sleep With the Angels, I'll Not Go Quietly*

Sometimes My Heart Goes Numb

Sometimes My Heart Goes Numb

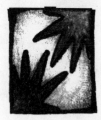

Love and Caregiving in a Time of AIDS

CHARLES GARFIELD

ORIGINATOR OF THE SHANTI MODEL USED WORLDWIDE

WITH CINDY SPRING & DORIS OBER

JOSSEY-BASS PUBLISHERS • SAN FRANCISCO

Substantial discounts on bulk quantities of Jossey-Bass books are available to corporations, professional associations, and other organizations. For details and discount information, contact the special sales department at Jossey-Bass Inc., Publishers. (415) 433–1740; FAX (800) 605-2665.

For sales outside the United States, please contact your local Paramount Publishing International Office.

 Manufactured in the United States of America on Lyons Falls Pathfinder Tradebook. This paper is acid-free and 100 percent totally chlorine-free.

Library of Congress Cataloging-in-Publication Data

Garfield, Charles A.
    Sometimes my heart goes numb : love and caregiving in a time of AIDS
/ by Charles A. Garfield with Cindy Spring and Doris Ober. — 1st ed.
       p.   cm. — (Jossey-Bass health series)
    Includes index.
    ISBN 0-7879-0105-9 (alk. paper)
    1. Shanti Project (San Francisco, Calif.) 2. AIDS (Disease)—
Patients—Care. I. Spring, Cindy. II. Ober, Doris. III. Title.
IV. Series V. Series: Jossey-Bass health series.
RC607.A26G36   1995
362.1'99792—dc20

                                      95-16261
                                         CIP

FIRST EDITION
HB Printing 10 9 8 7 6 5 4 3 2 1

Also by Charles Garfield:

BOOKS

Second to None: The Productive Power of Putting People First

Peak Performers

Peak Performance

*Stress and Survival: The Emotional Realities of
Life-Threatening Illness*

Psychosocial Care of the Dying Patient

Rediscovery of the Body: A Psychosomatic View of Life and Death

Consciousness: East and West (COAUTHOR)

AUDIOTAPE

AIDS Caregiving: Lessons for the Second Decade
(AVAILABLE FROM IMPACT AIDS IN SAN FRANCISCO)

To the thousands of Shanti Project

volunteers past and present.

For your courage to care

and for serving those who need you

with skill and compassion.

The moment we cease to hold each other,
the moment we break faith with one another
the sea engulfs us and the light goes out.

JAMES BALDWIN from *Loneliness and Love*
by Clark Moustakas

Nonetheless, he knew that the tale he had to tell could not be one of a final victory. It could be only the record of what had had to be done, and what assuredly would have to be done again in the never ending fight against terror and its relentless onslaughts, despite their personal afflictions, by all who, while unable to be saints but refusing to bow down to pestilences, strive their utmost to be healers.

ALBERT CAMUS, *The Plague*

The real meaning of suffering discloses itself only to him who has learned the art of compassion . . . gradually he will fall silent, and in the end will sit there wordless, for a long time sunk deep in himself. And the strange thing is that this silence is not felt by the other person as indifference, as a desolate emptiness which disturbs rather than calms. It is as if this silence had more meaning than countless words could ever have. It is as if he were being drawn into a field of force from which fresh strength flows into him. He feels suffused with a strange confidence. . . .

EUGEN HERRIGEL, *The Method of Zen*

It is true that these mysteries are dreadful, and people have always drawn away from them. But where can we find any-thing sweet and glorious that would never wear this mask of the dreadful? Whoever does not, some time or other, . . . give his full consent, his full and joyous consent to the dreadfulness of life, can never take possession of the unutterable abundance and power of our existence; can only walk on its edge, and one day, when the judgment is given, will have been neither alive nor dead.

RAINER MARIA RILKE, from a letter to Countess
Crouy, April 1923

Contents

Part One: A Communion of Caregivers

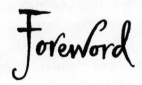

Foreword

I had seen Bill try it all. From God to science, through hell and back. His was a quest for finding peace in his dying time. Finally, in 1982, it was a Shanti-trained volunteer from San Francisco who gave him a few tools that would enable him to find that peace.

The week before he died, Bill asked me to visit him. We sat together on his front porch, which was dripping with wisteria, and he seemed almost spirit-like. I could see that his pain and struggle was, indeed, over. This was a man whose soul shone through his eyes. He asked me to promise to start an agency like Shanti in Los Angeles. He told me "nothing has meant more to me than the support I've gotten from my Shanti volunteer."

I promised, having no idea what I was getting into. In retrospect, Bill's death was the beginning of my journey to fulfill my heart's desire, a journey to serve others and to discover myself.

Later, some gifted caregivers came from San Francisco to teach us Shanti's philosophy and to provide us with a model for building a caregiving project based on open and honest communication. After our week-long training, I had more questions than when I started. That's when I met Charlie Garfield, Shanti Project's founder and long-term director, who had for years helped provide services to patients and loved ones facing life-challenging illnesses.

Charlie was living in the San Francisco Bay area, but made himself available to us then and over the years to answer our questions and to translate Shanti's essential components—nurturance and compassion without judgment—into skills that became our volunteers' strongest assets. He has done the same for many similar organizations around the world. Modeled after the original Shanti Project in San Francisco, Shanti Los Angeles has become a vital part of that city's health care community.

＿＿＿

In my decade of service, and since my own illness began, I've come to see both sides of caregiving. Caregiving is one way for humans to learn about humanity. It is not only about simply doing for others. It's also about self-acceptance and honest intentions. The best caregivers are those who come to the work not out of guilt or professional necessity, but because they have been touched by the soul of another human being.

Those are the people you'll meet in these pages. There is sadness and suffering in their stories, but more important, there is life in its true and raw form. As one caregiver put it, this work is "as real as it gets." As I write this piece in the shadow of my own death, my face and head covered with KS[1], I can honestly say that AIDS caregiving is also as profoundly enriching as it gets. In the compassionate world of caregiving, I experience these men and women as my brothers and sisters.

[1] See Glossary for definition.

June 1993   Daniel Warner
                                              Former Director
                                              L.A. Shanti

Sometimes
My Heart
Goes Numb

Introduction
Anatomy of a Mission

> The friend who can be silent with us in a moment of despair or confusion, who can stay with us in an hour of grief and bereavement, who can tolerate not knowing, not healing, not curing, and face with us the reality of our powerlessness, that is the friend who cares.
>
> —Henri J. Nouwen, *Out of Solitude*

Early in my clinical work at the University of California Medical Center, I sat at the bedside of a thirty-eight-year-old man who would die of his disease several days later. He had asked me to read to him from a book on his bedside table. It was the *Pensées*—the opposite of light reading—by the seventeenth-century French philosopher, Pascal. I read slowly; Roger seemed to doze, drifting in and out of waking-state consciousness, and I wondered if he heard me at all. Then suddenly, his eyes opened and he turned his head toward me. "Please read that again," he said. "The last line."

I repeated, "'The eternal silence of those infinite spaces frightens me.'"

Tears came to Roger's eyes, and he asked me to read it again, and then again. And then he said, with the tears brimming over and what I can only describe as relief in his voice, "Will you tell them—the doctors, the nurses—that *that's* why I'm so afraid."

I was a psychologist who specialized in helping cancer patients cope with the daily challenges of survival. And yet never had the distance between the healthy and the dying seemed so wide, so poignant, and so intolerable to me as when Roger found the words that enunciated his dread of the "eternal silence."

My regret was deep that I hadn't anticipated Roger's terror, and that I had only been able to offer him the words to express it by accident. But I was already learning that I was not the only member of what we like to think of as the healing professions whose healing skills left something to be desired.

Roger[1] was one of hundreds of patients who taught me that many of the psychological, social, and spiritual needs of people with life-threatening illnesses are seldom met in large medical institutions—not because medical professionals don't care, but because the resources, time, and training for these areas of caregiving are so limited. There is the notion within some medical institutions that staff training in other-than-physical caregiving is unnecessary, that such caregiving is basically hand-holding, or that medical professionals don't need seminars or class time in their already overcrowded days and nights for that sort of thing. And so, for emotional and psychological support, most patients must rely on compassionate friends, family members, and others in the same boat.

It was in addressing the need for a more holistic kind of caregiving on a broader, community level that I found a personal mission.

✦✦✦✦

In 1974 the clinical director of the cancer institute where I worked asked me to take a more active role in monitoring the psychosocial needs of our patients.

"What sort of caseload are we talking about?" I asked.

"Why, *all* of them," he said, surprised.

We had forty or fifty patients at the time, all facing the same "silences and spaces" that Roger had confronted. In varying degrees, each one needed attention, or conversation, or advocacy, or acknowledgment. Each one could easily occupy many hours or even whole days of my counsel and company.

"And I'd like you to think about psychosocial training sessions for the nursing staff," the director said, "and for our interns, as necessary."

The director may have been dreaming as far as reasonable goals are concerned, but I was inspired, especially about promoting patients' emotional, social, and psychological needs to their nurses and physicians. And then I thought, "why not in the larger community? Maybe we could offer services to ill people at home, too."

I couldn't get it out of my mind. Managing the hospital assignment—as well as my research and teaching—as best I could, I began to talk about a community-based system for meeting the other-than-physical needs of people with life-threatening illnesses. I talked to my students, to professional colleagues, to my family, to friends. We talked about office space, fund-raising events, salaries, staff—none of which we could afford and all foreign to me, a mathematician and psychologist by training, not a businessman.

What we could afford in the beginning was a single telephone number that people could call for information or help. And we could call on a resource that we hardly knew the breadth of—an army of people who cared.

We put out the word for volunteers, and we began screening those respondents and training them to give emotional and psychosocial support to people with life-threatening illnesses, mainly cancer, using an approach that I had developed at the Cancer Research Institute at the University of California. We also offered a matching service for patients and peer support volunteers. Without thinking, in a rapid response to a reporter's question, I called the project Shanti, a Sanskrit word that means "the peace that surpasses all understanding," or more succinctly, inner peace. This was the kind of peace that volunteers would find invaluable, and often in short supply, as their work increased.

Clearly, Shanti Project filled a void. Our meager press release, announcing our phone number and inviting calls, gained massive media attention, and the word spread. Over the next seven years, Shanti connected thousands of people facing life-threatening cancers with volunteers who served them with emotional support and as helping hands. By the end of the decade, more than three hundred organizations worldwide had contacted us about starting a community agency or hospital-based program modeled after Shanti Project.

By 1981, when what was referred to as "gay-related cancer" first appeared, Shanti was the first community-based agency of its kind in the country to respond. Since then many thousands of Shanti volunteers have stood by many more thousands of people living with AIDS, and in the past fourteen years, hundreds more people in similar projects have inquired about setting up services based on what became known as the Shanti model of peer support—a model born of necessity during my work at the bedside of patients like Roger.

It is from among those particular caregivers who have served during the AIDS days that I've drawn the cast of characters that occupies the following pages. They come from varied ethnic, cultural, and educational backgrounds, and are of different ages and sexual orientations. They are lovers, friends, family, volunteers, medical and mental health professionals, and clergy. They face the same fears and exhaustion and exhilaration as the previous generation of caregivers did—but because it's AIDS, they also face unprecedented challenges.

I saw a client at the hospital and said goodbye to him. When I say goodbye, I mean this person's going to be dead— I'll never see him again. Two weeks later, I saw him at the mall. AIDS is such a roller coaster. You just don't know.
                                    —Penny Chernow, Marin AIDS Project

The difficulty in predicting what will happen next to a person with AIDS is one of the disease's most insidious aspects. When constant change is the norm, caregivers must plan for uncertainty rather than for a predictable next stage of the illness. And uncertainty exacerbates the feeling of inadequacy that is the bane of caregivers, perhaps even more so among physicians and nurses, who are accustomed to exactitude and taught to project a semblance of self-assuredness.

Because AIDS as we know it is a relatively new phenomenon, the amount of literature available on it, though growing fast, is far less daunting than the volumes that exist on many other types of life-threatening diseases, like certain kinds of cancer, for instance. Many people with AIDS (and many Shanti volunteers) have kept up with the constantly expanding fund of data on the disease. While shifting opinions on treatment, prognosis, and the course of the illness can cause confusion and anxiety, it is not uncommon for the patient who monitors the latest breaking news on the disease to be better informed than his caregiver or even his physician, a phenomenon I believe to be unprecedented in medicine, and one that requires a great deal of humility, flexibility, and willingness to collaborate on the part of all parties.

AIDS comes not only with its terrible spectrum of physical insults, but with a social stigma not attached to most other illnesses. Society's condemnation can be devastating to its recipients, and caregivers must have special sensitivity to their patient's level of self-esteem, and sometimes their piercing feelings of guilt for having contracted the disease. And in an odd application of "guilt by association," more than one AIDS caregiver has felt the sting of social and even professional disapproval for working with people with AIDS.

Unlike most other caregivers, people who care for people with AIDS sometimes find themselves engaged in decision making or consultations with extended gay families, which may include a life-long partner, lovers, friends, parents, and children. Sometimes a caregiver must console parents long absent from their son's life, who have been called to a hospital in a strange city only to learn for the first time that their son is homosexual, and that he is dying of a disease they may never be able to mention to their neighbors. And there are unique ethical issues that come up now and then—conflicts between a patient's biological family and his lover, for instance—in which the caregiver may have to mediate, or act as the patient's advocate, or from which he or she may have to protect the patient.

Another challenge quite specific to AIDS caregiving exists among those people with AIDS who are intravenous drug users. In addition to their illness, these folks may be dealing with addiction, homelessness, and hunger. For some of them a diagnosis of AIDS is secondary to where their next fix or their baby's next meal will come from. For them, medical bills and miracle cures are not as compelling as housing, food stamps, and drug treatments. These clients are frequently African-American and Hispanic people whose needs are quite different from the middle-class gay white men who brought AIDS to the attention of the nation. For the caregiver, it may be a whole new world with a whole new set of rules and priorities. One exasperated counselor told me, "Some of these people are sleeping on cardboard out in the street, and the doctor expects them to have their pills all lined up and organized, and to take them at one o'clock. It's a joke."

While gay and bisexual men with AIDS have certain specific needs in coping with their illness, and IV drug users have certain others, women with AIDS, especially those with children, may face a whole other set of circumstances and require a whole different kind of help from their caregivers.

Neuropsychiatric complications—short-term memory loss, disorientation, hallucination, depression, erratic behavior—are all common afflictions among people with AIDS, which presents another challenge to caregivers. One AIDS counselor who cared for a patient with dementia-related hallucinations told me he has learned to let go of literal interpretations and to "listen between the lines" for his patient's meaning.

AIDS caregivers must also factor into their efforts the fact that along with their health, their clients have frequently lost their entire support system—dozens or even hundreds of friends and acquaintances—to the disease. These clients may be quite devastatingly alone. And companionship is only part of what they may have given up. Losses include sexuality, intimate relationships, one's looks, job, independence, and self-esteem. Protracted grief may be the most constant companion of a person with AIDS.

> I've been supporting people with AIDS for over ten years now, and I think if you do anything over and over again, you learn how to do it well. What passes in the world for tragedies happen every day. I hear about them, I see them. I can't be knocked against the wall by each one. I have to construct a coping technique that allows me to survive and also offer the most compassion and love that I can.
>
> —Carol Kleinmaier, support group coordinator

Most of the caregivers you will meet in these pages have been on the front lines of the AIDS pandemic for many years. Like combat soldiers in fierce wars, and not unlike the very people they care for, they too have experienced many losses in a relatively brief period of time, and they never feel absolutely sure they've done enough. Sometimes their hearts go numb, which is a fact of life for long-term caregivers—a fact captured by caregiver Wayne Corbitt in the poem that opens his chapter and that inspired our book's title. Many AIDS-generation caregivers risk the same traumatic stress syndrome that occurs among veterans of bloody wars; but many others have learned self-care strategies to cope with "compassion fatigue," self-doubt, and fear.

Caregivers spoke to us candidly about the toughest parts of the job, about choices and situations that had no obvious solutions, about feelings of hopeless inadequacy. Yet some of these same experiences become turning points for our subjects, vastly extending feelings of self-esteem, and clearly enhancing their effectiveness as caregivers.

Furthermore, these friends and lovers and volunteers and clergy and nurses and doctors reported almost unanimously that they could see their care making a difference. "Healing" occurred, even though it wasn't necessarily physical healing. (By *healing*, we mean restoration of wholeness in its broadest sense. On the physical level, healing refers to a restoration of function and the end of pain. Healing can also occur on psychological, emotional, and spiritual levels as well. These include an end to addictions, depression, anxiety, terror, estrangement from loved ones, and feelings of isolation and disconnection.) And this healing doesn't just happen for the person with AIDS. Our caregivers discovered it was happening for them as well. Every compassionate soul whom you will meet in these pages had some significant personal wound when he or she began caring for someone else. These were wounds sustained in childhood or adulthood or both. Some caregivers had been acutely abused; others had been hurt in ways that were chronic and less obvious. In many cases, in trying to heal their respective wounds, these caregivers were drawn, consciously or not, to healing others.

I would never say that personal pain is always a prerequisite to effective caregiving, nor that AIDS caregivers are attracted to the work primarily because they desire to lessen their own suffering. But I do say that the exemplary caregivers whose stories you will read here have learned a great deal from their own pain about themselves and about how to best care for the people they serve.

Swiss psychiatrist Carl Jung called such people "Wounded Healers," and asserted that in the relationship between caregiver and patient, the two roles transcend one another. The wounded healer recognizes himself or herself in the patient, and the patient recognizes his or her reflection in the healer. Both caregiver and patient step through the looking glass, in a manner of speaking, and into the territory of the other. Ancient healers, shamans, believed that this ability to move "between the worlds" of health and sickness was the source of their powers to heal.

Shanti counselor Bharat Lindemood fell headlong into that place between worlds when he first started working with AIDS patients in San Francisco General Hospital's Ward 5A. He recalled:

I went into the room of a man who was very far along in AIDS dementia. He was pretty incoherent most of the time. He was in bed under the covers, with his head buried under the pillow. I said his name softly, and introduced myself as a Shanti counselor. He peeked out at me from under the pillow and said, "Come back later when I can help you."

It was a moment of lucidity for him, like a crack in the sidewalk. I was so stunned that it took me a minute to digest what he'd said. Then I stammered out something like, "Wait . . . You don't understand . . . I'm here to help you . . ." But he was gone, buried under his pillow again.

The patient's identification with the healing capacities of the caregiver can provide an unexpected source of strength for the patient, triggering a kind of internal tap on his or her healing resources. Ultimately, for the wounded healer, the act of giving is also one of gaining, as the stories that follow make clear.

It was true for Chuck Landis, a vice-president at the Bank of America in San Francisco when his partner, Ed, was diagnosed with AIDS in 1987. Chuck told me:

I made a commitment on the spot that I was going to go through this with him. And I remember Ed saying, "Do you know what you're letting yourself in for?" And I said, "Yes, of course I do." And yes, of course I didn't. I had no idea. At the time it made no difference what we were getting ourselves into, we were going to go through whatever he went through together.

I didn't know it then, but I know it now that my caregiving experience with him on a very personal, twenty-four-hour-a-day, four-year duration was the most human, the most profound thing I've ever done in my life.

We have allowed our caregivers to speak for themselves as much as possible, about their roles in relationship to their clients and patients, about the rewards they've received in the course of their most compassionate service, and about everything else—the kinds of resources they brought with them to the job, what has helped and what hasn't, what they've feared and what they've overcome, and what they have learned by way of practical skills that can be used by family members, professionals, and volunteers in any home, hospital, or agency where caregivers work or live with people with AIDS as well as with other patient populations.

Our caregivers offer their stories as a kind of evidence. They are teaching tales in a narrative form, a form that psychology, psychiatry, nursing, and other human disciplines are beginning to recognize as a legitimate approach to unearthing some essential truths. Now that many of Shanti's finest caregivers have taken important positions in other AIDS organizations, and have carried their teaching tales with them, those truths are traveling far and wide. The Shanti model, as reflected in these stories, has moved beyond a single organization in San Francisco, one that is changing dramatically. Shanti, like other AIDS agencies, tries to carry on in an era of shrinking resources, but its model is alive and well within the many organizations whose caregiving activities have been informed and inspired by it.

Many of the caregivers' stories in this book reflect the terminal reality in which they live and work, a milieu in which the truth is that, so far, most people diagnosed with AIDS die. Nevertheless, these caregivers maintain a life-affirming partnership with their loved ones or clients or patients. For all of them, support is the principal caregiving task: supporting the client's or patient's or loved one's efforts to live with AIDS; and should death approach, supporting that person in his or her dying time.

The caregiver who has given up on the client's possibility for survival, or whose words or actions undercut, however subtly, a client's will to live, seriously jeopardizes the healing partnership with that person. Such a caregiver may actually be a danger to the person with AIDS, sabotaging his or her efforts to survive in relatively good health with the disease, as many do—in many cases for many years. People with AIDS deserve every bit as much supportive caregiving in their fight for life as those who are dying do at the end of their days.

Michael Callen was a survivor who lived twelve years with AIDS. He wrote in words I'll never forget about his personal struggle: "I have railed against, and cursed, and challenged hopelessness wherever I have encountered it," he said. "Believing that I could survive is probably the precondition necessary for my survival."[2] Imagine if you were Michael Callen, and your caregiver didn't believe deep down that you could survive. How could he or she fully support you then?

I suspect that our caregivers' strong commitment to support their clients' efforts to live well with AIDS, and even survive the illness altogether, may be not only practical, but visionary. Each of us is rooting for the day when the notion of surviving AIDS is a commonplace reality. The comparatively new discipline of psychoneuroimmunology may help us to understand whether a mind/body link is basic to surviving AIDS. In related research, Lisa Berkman, an epidemiologist and public health specialist at the Yale Medical School, found that friendless patients die at three times the rate after a heart attack than others who have family or friends to help them recover.[3] If it turns out that survival is linked with psychosocial factors as well as physical ones such as the functioning of the immune system, then the life-affirming attitudes and actions of caregivers may be even more valuable than we have suspected all along.

◆ ◆ ◆

The people you'll read about in this book, and thousands like them around the world, are the heart of AIDS caregiving. To those of our readers who may be caring or anticipating caring for someone with AIDS, our message to you is that you are not alone. For here are some of the legions of men and women no braver than yourself, with much to share, who are with you.

Notes

1. The names of care recipients in this book have been changed to protect their privacy.

2. Michael Callen, "I Will Survive," *Village Voice*, May 3, 1988, pp. 34–35.

3. Berkman's study of nearly two hundred older men and women found that 53 percent died within six months if they had no close personal sources of support, compared with 36 percent with one source, and 23 percent with two or more people to care for them. (Charles Petit, "Love May Heal Heart Patients," *San Francisco Chronicle*, Jan. 19, 1995, p. A14.)

Part One

A Communion of Caregivers

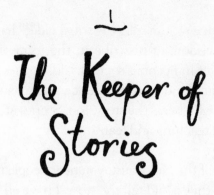

The Keeper of Stories

Eric Shifler was motivated to become a Shanti volunteer "partly by fear, partly wanting to help, partly out of anger, and partly having a roommate real sick. It was that crisis mentality—no one else was going to help us, we had to do it ourselves."

Eric's roommate had been diagnosed with Kaposi's sarcoma in 1981, before AIDS even had a name. Eric was diagnosed HIV+ in 1985. That year he joined the Shanti staff as a volunteer coordinator.

Because I was in it since the beginning of the epidemic,
I feel like a walking archive sometimes. Like a tribal elder.
But I would rather belong to a different tribe, if you know
what I mean.

    The hard part is you have to live with so many memories
of people who are dead. What I like about it is the giving.
You get to give your knowledge, you get to train someone
to do peer counseling, or to give unconditional support and
love. One thing I've learned is if you have the experience,
if you have the knowledge, if you care, it doesn't do any good
unless you give it to the people out there who need it.

Eric's reference to himself as a "tribal elder" has to do with his collecting the wisdom of his tribe in the form of stories, as the senior members of indigenous societies do. Stories allow the teller to express emotion and gain coherence and meaning, and this is true for the one who hears the story, too. Stories are the traditional medium of both teaching and learning.

In accounts of the Holocaust, you hear people talk about surviving so they could tell the story. I have all these memories now, all these stories, and I help people with AIDS and their families and friends and lovers survive to tell theirs.

Keeping the stories in his memory, and sharing them with others is consistent with Eric's vision of himself as a walking archive. And it affirms a common theme among caregivers—the importance of and the value in bearing witness. Telling the stories of individuals with AIDS—and of individual caregivers—is another way of keeping the ones we've lost alive, as much as it is a chronicle or documentary of an especially awful disease.

Essential to his role as an archivist is Eric's skill at "active listening," which is listening from the heart, without judgment, to the stories of those he cares for. Eric knows that such listening has healing properties. He knows that living with AIDS is sometimes like living in a pressure cooker, and that sometimes you have to let off steam or you think you'll explode. He knows that some people are desperate to talk—to tell their stories—and that when people are grieving they may need to repeat their stories over and over.

Letting our stories out, revealing our secrets, our joys, our sorrows, is a way of defining ourselves and describing our journeys, a way we show that we are unique. Letting our stories out is a way we begin to understand our struggles and reconcile them. It may also be a painful process. When the story comes wrenching out from some long-buried place inside, it reveals both pain and unresolved conflict—and it hurts to tell it. And for the listener, when the story's moral or its conclusion is not one we want to hear—it hurts

to hear it. Eric tells the story of a homophobic father that demonstrates this point.

I'd been working as a counselor on San Francisco General
Hospital's Ward 5A [also referred to as the AIDS Ward]
with a patient who was very nervous because his family was
coming. His mother knew he was gay but the father didn't,
and he was going to tell the father.

So the parents came, they went into the room, and about
a half hour later, the father comes storming out. I introduced
myself and asked if there was anything I could do, and he
just went off, raving about faggots and his faggot son and
God's punishment and all of that.

I validated what he was saying. I said, "Yes, it must be
horrible to have a gay son when society says it's wrong."

I felt helpless because I wanted to listen to the man,
but I also wanted to slap him upside the head and tell him,
"Buddy, what's happening here is bigger than the stereotypes
you're holding onto. Your son is dying." But I knew I wasn't
there to debate him on the pros and cons of being gay. I was
there to provide support, and that meant letting him vent
his anger about gayness. I managed to not put my agenda
on him.

When the father found out later that I was gay, he was
mortified. I saw him the next day and he wouldn't look at
me, so I went up to him and I told him that what he had
said yesterday—I knew he had to say those things. He didn't
have to feel sorry about anything. If it helped him with his
son, that was fine. And the man was just dumbfounded.

But he wouldn't go back into his son's room. I think it
was a combination of gay and AIDS and grief. He never
would go back in that room.

Living in the crucible of the AIDS pandemic causes all of us to
exhibit less than our best behavior at times. Eric excuses shabby

behavior when it's a secondary concern, and works hard to show that he's aware of how difficult it is for his clients and their loved ones to live with AIDS. But it takes a while to achieve the equanimity one needs to listen to this father's homophobia, and to understand that people with AIDS and their families may be living in a turmoil of emotions that can exacerbate weak or damaged connections among family members.

A less experienced caregiver might act out his own emotional response to the father's words, might not be able to resist the negative reaction. A less experienced caregiver might not have understood that the father's anger was his way of defending himself against the shock and terror of learning that his son had AIDS, was gay, and was dying. In Eric's case, his composure and restraint are particularly admirable because he surely heard the echo of his own father's anger and disgust in the voice of the father who could not be with his son.

◢ ◢ ◢

Eric was raised in a small coal mining town north of Scranton, Pennsylvania, in the 1950s and 1960s. He recalled the first discussion of his homosexuality:

> I announced I was "queer"—that's what it was called then—over a Sunday dinner when I was six or seven. I'd been playing ball with a bunch of kids and some guy walked by and one of the older kids said, "That guy's queer." I asked what that meant and they told me. I had already been doing all that stuff, so I knew I was queer too. I didn't know that it was bad, though, nobody said that.
>
> So at dinner I announced that I was queer, and the mashed potatoes went flying. I remember my father hit me, but he was an alcoholic, so that wasn't unusual. Slappings, locked in the bedroom. Winter time, locked outside. There was lots of physical abuse from him.

Later, everyone in high school also knew I was gay.
I remember walking into a classroom and having the entire
class holler, "Homo!" A teacher called me queer one time.
I never forgot that. That kind of wounding made me more
open to other people's pain.

So I've been yelled at before. And not only in my distant
past, but from walking down the street on Tuesday. You get
called "faggot" from a car; someone yells, "AIDS carrier!"
It's nothing I haven't heard at least a hundred times already.
It's lost its shock value.

The words have lost their power to shock, and Eric has gained
a perspective that takes precedence over the question of whose
truth to defend. More important than debate in the case of the
homophobic father was minimizing conflicts and resolving differences. And for Eric, this is an unanticipated psychological boon.
In choosing not to go head to head with the raging father, but to let
the man's offensive words sail by, Eric chooses not to be a target.
Eric's stance is one of flexibility and tolerance. In a way, his tolerance puts him out of the line of this father's fire, and retroactively,
out of the line of his own father's rage. From this position it is possible to forgive the homophobic father, and indirectly his own
father, for their hostility.

By his example, Eric teaches us to choose our battles. There are
some things he might have argued about in other times and different places that are not worth struggling over now. He "would have
responded very differently" to the father who would not be with
his son had they met outside of Eric's work, he told me; but his primary agenda in supporting his client was to create a safe, peaceful
environment for him, and even for his father. "The trick is,"
according to Eric, "to leave your agenda at the door. You can
always pick it up when you leave. When you go into a client's
home or into a patient's room, you're there to hear their story, not
to tell them yours."

We come back to the value of hearing the stories of the ones we care for, even when the tales test our emotional, psychological, and spiritual resources. These difficult stories may trigger quantum leaps into greater emotional strength and compassion for those we serve. If we can reach past our fear or anger about what we are hearing, and maintain our supportive presence rather than defend our feelings or rush in with advice or offer a rebuttal, then we can be of real service.

Listening is the single strongest asset a caregiver can bring to this work. Active listening makes the listener a participant in another person's drama and requires a willingness to walk into the emotional life of that person when invited to do so, to be there for another as fully and consciously as we can, to share the client's hopes and fears. For when we listen, we are helping the storyteller. When we listen we are giving of ourselves. Listening is how we learn, and how we connect with the teller. Such connection is precisely what Eric did not have and could not get, at least from his father, as he grew up. Fortunately for those he works with, Eric's isolation created in him a need to give what he had lacked; he feels charged to be an audience for others.

✐ ✐ ✐

Sometimes I let families know right away that I'm gay. I say something like, "It must be very difficult for you to be in this situation, knowing that I and other people here are gay—but I want you to know we're here to help you, so if you need anything, I want you to ask me." And I'm saying to myself, "Before you leave here, you'll know that I'm more than just gay—you'll know that I'm a care provider. You'll know that I would help you any way I could." Your ego comes into it. You want to show them that you're more than they think you are.

Eric discovered that being gay had a positive, life-affirming side when he moved to New York: "I spent my twenties and early thirties there. It was magical. It was the 1970s in Greenwich Village, and gay liberation." Eric became an X-ray technician. He was especially interested in head injuries and worked at an acute care trauma center in Manhattan for several years. It was basic training for the AIDS pandemic.

My work revolved around life-threatening injuries—an auto accident, a brain tumor. The work didn't frighten me. The epidemic frightens me still, but doing the work—no. My work then was understanding that this person is nervous about this test, or the person's family is, and being able to assure them that "I'm with you, and we can get through this together." I never felt I was doing anything special. I just had to do whatever was necessary to get the X-rays.

So today if one of the patients on the ward is having a test, I know he's scared. The doctors want to do a bone marrow biopsy, and the patients freak. But because of my medical background, I can talk them through it. I can relate to the doctors who have to get the test done, and the patients who have the test done to them.

Eric's ability to relate to people on both sides of a shared situation, like doctor and patient, makes him as sensitive to the needs and concerns of the family and friends of a person with AIDS as he is to the person himself. He has helped parents cope with the sometimes shocking revelation that their child is gay, or an intravenous drug user, or is dying.

Sometimes loved ones arrive at San Francisco General Hospital from far away, knowing no one, with no place to stay. Because San Francisco General is a public hospital, its patients may be indigent, and visiting parents may have only minimal resources themselves.

I remember this woman who came from New Jersey to see her daughter. All she knew was that her daughter was very sick and had been taken to the hospital. She arrived at San

Francisco General with her suitcase in her hand two hours after her daughter had died. I was there when the nurse told her, and the woman collapsed. She just crumpled to the floor.

We took her to the Shanti office on the floor, and I sat with her for about three hours in a grief counseling session. We talked about what a wonderful person the daughter had been, and how terrible that this could happen. She was raw. I just sat and listened to her ramble, listened to her vent her feelings.

Then she realized she had no place to stay. She had, I think, twenty-eight dollars in her pocket. I got her a place at the Family Link. I helped her make the funeral arrangements, because she couldn't afford to have the body taken back to New Jersey.

She didn't know anyone else in the city, and for the next three or four days I got at least two calls from this woman a day. She'd say, "I didn't sleep last night," so we'd talk about that. Whatever went on. In between, I'd be running from room to room dealing with other people, so I'd just catch it as I could, go with whatever she was talking about for a while, until she calmed down.

Pain may tumble through a barrage of words in rambling remembrances. Sometimes compulsive chatter, mundane and seemingly inconsequential discussions help smooth and soften feelings that are too sharp to handle. For some people, even usually taciturn individuals, the rush of words comes unbidden, naturally, a survival skill that we didn't know we had. Others need help, need a receptive listener to acknowledge their suffering; need a nod or comment to encourage them to continue, to go on talking it out.

Eric pointed out that in the whirlwind of an epidemic, doctors, nurses, and even social workers seldom have time to devote to real listening, at least not the time required. "They're always running," Eric said, "whereas in our job, that's what we're there for. To sit and listen."

There was a young man I met when he was first diagnosed with PCP a couple of years ago, and I saw him through the course of his illness. I knew there was something in his past. He had said there was something he couldn't tell anybody.

The week before he died he was real sick, and he called me. When I went to see him he let it all out that he'd been caught stealing to support his drug habit, and gone to prison, and been raped in prison. And after he talked about what it was like being raped, he was calmer for the next several days. I think he was able to tell me because he knew whatever he said wasn't going to blow me out of the water, and he could trust me.

Being able to hear anything and everything and not be "blown out of the water," is one of the tasks of a tribal elder, at least in the large tribe of those who have been affected by AIDS. The listener is not asked to judge, and certainly not condemn; he or she need not offer absolution. Active listening is done with the heart. The active listener acknowledges that what he or she hears is true for the teller. This is not such an easy task. Novice caregivers frequently find it takes many clients and years of practice to suspend judgments, biases, and prejudices to listen from the heart.

✎ ✎ ✎

Mania can be a way of responding to fear. Acknowledgment is sometimes the only comfort a caregiver can offer in these situations, but sometimes acknowledgment doesn't help and there is simply nothing you can do.

It was the first time I was with someone who didn't die peacefully. Usually they're snowed with morphine or something. But this man was on nothing and he was manic. "Straighten this up, put this here, do this, do that . . ."—all in the hour before he died. I didn't know how to handle him. I didn't know how to be in that situation. I know now it's okay to be manic. It's okay to do whatever you're going to do. Not that I have to get manic with you, but I have to let you be manic. If you want me to straighten a stack of papers, I will, but I'll say, "This is horrible for me—what must it be like for you?"

But at the time I had this patient, I was nowhere near doing that. Now when I go to see someone, the first thing I do is to check where they're at—whether they're escalating, or depressed, or anxious. I don't get anxious with them, but I understand that they are that way and I let them be that way. I don't try to fix it. I don't say, "You'll be okay," or "This won't take long." They may not be, and it may. I just try to be there, wherever they're at.

"Wherever they're at" may be a frightening place. "Being there" means being there in context—sensing what your client is experiencing in the context of the disease and its assaults. A lot of otherwise "abnormal" behavior becomes understandable in the shadow AIDS casts. Eric cautions against labeling anyone's behavior abnormal.

I remember this man at General who had been diagnosed with depression, and the psych residents wanted to put him on all these meds, which he said made him drowsy. We Shanti counselors, social workers, and nurses were all thinking, "Here's a gay man in his late thirties who's lived in San Francisco since the early 1970s. AIDS started killing his friends in 1981. Now it's 1994 and just about everyone he ever knew in the city has died. Wouldn't you be depressed?"

We tried to explain this to the [doctors]. They aren't living in the midst of the epidemic. They think they are, but unless it's in your community, I don't think you get it that the real pathology is accumulated grief. Depression is not just that you've been diagnosed yourself, but that forty of your friends have also died, and it all adds up.

It's true that my professional colleagues sometimes forget what it means to be living in the world of AIDS. Behaviors that might not be "normal"—whatever that means—in daily life, become understandable when one considers the terrible stress associated with AIDS, and all the fears that go along with it. Chronic trauma is a frequent companion of AIDS, and otherwise strange behaviors, like a preoccupation with stories about the dead, make all the sense in the world when you take the scope and range of HIV disease into consideration.

Along with depression, we deal with frustration, and anger, and grief. Like other experienced caregivers, Eric relies on support groups and informal conversation with caregiving colleagues to keep on the upside of emotional overload. Training others to become peer counselors for people with AIDS is another way of modifying his frustrations in the work—a way Eric can "talk it out" for himself, and at the same time prepare the next generation of caregivers for their own challenging paths.

Humor is also a way he copes with frustration and tragedy, and gallows humor, which Freud considered one of the most mature forms of psychological defense, is Eric's means of lightening the often relentless seriousness of life in the world of AIDS. He told me the story of a patient with dementia, for instance, whom he observed pulling a toaster around by the cord. "He was just taking his toaster for a walk," Eric explained. "I told him to come right back and don't plug it in anywhere."

2

I See Miracles All the Time

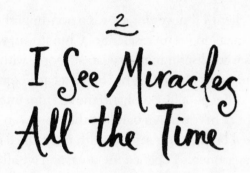

Those people who said I was different—who suggested
there was something wrong with me when I was growing
up—maybe some of them are smiling now, and saying,
"He's different, that's wonderful."

Danny Castelow has a rich baritone voice and a broad smile; he
moves with a dancer's grace. He is an exceptional man whose
approach to caregiving is distinguished by a profound level of
respect, acceptance, and validation of his clients with AIDS. He
tries to look at each one without prejudice and without assumptions. His special skill is astutely assessing his clients' individual
needs and going the extra mile to meet them. I asked him how he
learns about another person's needs.

It's not complicated. It's mainly just having a conversation
with someone with the intent of getting to know him or her.
It's realizing that just because you've worked with sixty other
people with AIDS who have had pneumocystis twice, you
may not have the least idea where this person with his second
bout is coming from. Every case and every client is unique.

One client I'll never forget was a non-English-speaking Asian man, a long-term resident of Chinatown, where the landlords were discriminating against people with AIDS. Where this man was living, he shared a bathroom with eighteen other people. So Shanti moved him into a small apartment of his own in a building they ran as an AIDS residence. I brought a translator with us on the day we showed him the apartment. I opened the door, and we all walked in.

I began telling the translator and the translator began telling him that there were some additional pieces of furniture in the basement that he could use, and he was waving his hand as if to say, "I don't want to hear. I don't even care about that now!" He was just basking in this empty apartment that was all his. And he was totally fixated on the bathroom! If we had only rented him that bathroom, I think he would have been thrilled. Seeing what it meant to him and realizing that I had played a little part in giving him something that was so important was one of the most incredible moments I've had in this work.

You try to honor individual needs. And that's not always going to be what your agency offers. Somebody might arrive at your office who should be across town. In the case of the Asian man, it took three agencies going beyond "what's on the menu," to get him his apartment.

I've made it a personal challenge to put people together with the agency or person who can help them. To do that I may try a little more, or try a different way. Instead of, "We don't do whatever it is," I'd rather say, "We don't do it, but here's the name and phone number of an agency that does."

Danny tries to go the distance for his clients precisely because he views each one as unique and deserving of his best effort. He is interested in who they are *now*, with AIDS and all its complications, which is a kind of validation that not only demonstrates respect for his clients, but encourages their self-respect—a precious commodity to someone with severe, self-eroding physical and emotional challenges. How his clients respond to those challenges is what touches and inspires Danny.

It was Ted's birthday on the day his doctors told him that he wouldn't be going home because his lover couldn't provide the kind of skilled care he was going to need from now on, and they were going to move him to a hospice.

When I stopped into his room that afternoon, his family was throwing him a party that had obviously been planned beforehand. There were balloons, some of his co-workers from his job were there, his lover was there, there was a cake and photographs of him when he was well. And the look on his face—well, he was just horrified.

I went back that evening, and said, "Your face didn't match what was happening this afternoon," and I could see him release and then he burst into tears and said, "I just want to go home."

It was one of those moments that you might want to turn away from, but I've learned to sort of hang out in those painful moments. People don't go into cardiac arrest when you tell them the truth. Ted had needed someone to acknowledge what was happening and how he felt—that he wasn't going to go home—and how sad that was.

But you have to learn that. You have to practice not turning away from the truth. It's easier to do what Ted's family and friends did. Six years ago, I would have been partying with them.

When Danny talks about "hanging out with pain" he is describing that kind of deep listening that is key to the Shanti model of caregiving. It requires intent listening to the client and to one's own intuition—and it requires not trying to do or to fix. It's a way of being fully present for another person and bearing witness to his or her struggle. It may also open the door to profound experiences:

> There was a patient at San Francisco General who had six-teen different AIDS-related infections. There wasn't room on his chart to write them all. At the time there were only twenty-two recognized by the CDC, and he had sixteen of them.
>
> This man had an incredible speaking voice, and perfect diction, and although he was very weak, he took great pleasure in reciting what he had: "I have toxoplasmosis, and cryptococcosis, and Kaposi's sarcoma, and cytomegalo-virus . . ." and on and on. I was inclined to cut him off, but I let him go through the whole list, which ended with him saying, "And you know, with all of these things that are happening to me, I can really say that I'm having a good life." Not "I've had a good life"—I'm having a good life.
>
> You have to be inspired by a person like that. After deal-ing with that kind of person, I have a hard time with small complaints. People say, "It must be so hard, AIDS work," but for me it's harder dealing with petty, non-AIDS related things.

While there are no formulas for responses or behaviors that we can pass on to future caregivers, we can try to advance the notion of being fully present, of letting go of trying to control things, and of trusting the process of caregiving and the very special something that can happen between two people in the caregiving relationship.

One way to let go and trust in the power of the caregiving rela-tionship is to have let go and learned to trust oneself. Danny pays attention to himself, he is introspective and committed to personal and professional growth. He told me quite sincerely, "I think deep in my heart I'm a very nice person with a wonderful, kind spirit. I work on cultivating that. You have to work on yourself. You have to be very conscious." His view of himself as a "kind spirit" is strongly supported by colleagues and clients.

- - - -

Danny has been very conscious, very sensitive, from childhood. He grew up in Detroit, and demonstrated a talent for dance at an early age, which was acknowledged, and nourished, and grew into a promising career. He toured with various dance and theater companies when he was in his twenties.

Danny had three sisters, one only fourteen months older, with whom he was especially close.

We were crazy about each other and spent all our time together as children. And then one day the lady across the street was outside cutting her hedges, and she caught me by myself and told me, "Danny, don't you play with your sister so much. A little boy shouldn't spend so much time with his sister." I was seven or eight.

Was the neighbor insinuating something incestuous between Danny and his sister, or was she warning him against becoming effeminate by spending too much time with her? Danny was clever enough, and sensitive enough to catch the subliminal criticism, even if the specifics were vague. It may have been the first time someone had said, in effect, "You're different, Danny Castelow. And we don't tolerate that difference."

For this sensitive boy, the comment was a slap, a resounding invalidation. But invalidation can occur far more subtly—it can consist of a simple discouraging word; it can be felt in a person's rolled eyes, in the projection of doubt: "Are you really sure you want to do that?" It comes through in innuendo. Danny believes, "If you're judgmental or skeptical about something, it's going to show."

At the same time his meddlesome neighbor was making Danny feel bad about himself and his loving relationship with his sister, he was going to dancing school, "and here the teachers told us, 'Lift your heads! You're beautiful! Don't you know you're the descendants of kings and queens of Africa?' " In the course of the day the messages Danny got and the way he was treated by the adults in his environment were quite inconsistent and oftentimes conflicting. "No wonder I was a mess!" he says.

> But so many of my clients have similar stories. Most people I've worked with get into childhood stuff at some point. I've had some tell me that they would rather their parents had physically abused them than to have ignored them, or dismissed them, or invalidated them as they had. I understand what they're saying: They wanted to be recognized for who they were, they needed to know they mattered.

They still do. And it was, and is, the same for Danny. But his encounter with invalidation seems to have made him vow never to be guilty of doing the same to someone else. His promise is, "I'll always try to see who the other person is, and what he or she needs, and I'll try not to put a negative slant on my view of that." He tries to do what his dance teachers did: to give the people he works with the gift of affirmation and pride.

*   *   *   *

Danny began his Shanti caregiving as a volunteer at the same time he was working for a fast-paced brokerage firm. Soon he traded one high-pressure job for another: in 1986 he joined the staff at Shanti and became director of Practical Support. Later he worked as a counselor at San Francisco General Hospital's Ward 5A, and then as case manager for Shanti House, a residence for people with AIDS. Today he is a case manager for the San Francisco AIDS Foundation. His evolution as a caregiver has been marked by profound lessons learned on the job.

> When I was a volunteer, most of my clients were wonderful. I've worked with people who would get up and clean their

apartment before I came over to clean it, so it would be less
of a burden on me. Then I got assigned a really mean man.
According to his friends, John had always been mean. But
I didn't know how to deal with it. I didn't know to trust the
same instincts that applied to nice clients—to tell the truth,
to be able to say what's going on for me.

One day when I got to John's after a particularly bad day
at work, he snapped at me about something, and I managed
to say, "Listen, this isn't working for me." And he said,
"You don't understand. I was taken to emergency today.
I've had a horrible day!" And suddenly it felt okay to say to
him, "You don't understand. I work for five stockbrokers and
they were all on my ass today, and I had a rotten day too!"

Then we sat down and told each other about our awful
days. It was really wonderful. If we hadn't gotten there, I
probably would have asked to be assigned to someone else.

John didn't get any nicer, and nothing seemed to change
with him, but I really enjoyed working with him afterward.
There was something very rich about sitting down and saying,
"Can we work together? What can we get done?"

There are also situations where the client isn't abusive, but the
circumstances are especially tough to deal with.

I was working with a man at Shanti House, who had such
extensive KS progression on his leg that the leg was literally
dead. The doctors had offered him amputation as an option,
but he thought as long as he could still walk on it he would
keep it. So every so often they took him into surgery and cut
away the dead skin, and a wound specialist visited him at his
apartment three times a day.

I also met with him at his apartment, and it was the
hardest thing I ever had to deal with, because of the smell of
decomposing flesh. He would be talking to me and I couldn't

really hear him—much of the time I was fighting not to vomit. And I could see that he was aware of it too, and very uncomfortable about it.

The sad part was that he was such an amazing man. He was a schoolteacher and had been teacher-of-the-year several times, and all the kids loved him. He was very engaging, very energetic, yet his leg stood in the way of everything.

I cried over this. It wasn't something a support group or the Shanti House director could get me through. I had fantasies about convincing him to have the leg amputated. I imagined what it was like for him when he took a taxi to make his doctor's appointments, or when he sat down next to someone in the waiting room at San Francisco General. I imagined everyone had the same reaction as me.

But then the woman would come—the wound care specialist—three times a day to unwrap this leg and dress it and come back later. I thought this was totally amazing. There was something in her powerful enough to move past this overwhelmingly unpleasant thing to do her job. I drew the strength to go back and see him from her.

The last time I saw him was my last day at Shanti House. He had asked me to come up to say goodbye. I braced myself and walked in—and there was no odor! The wound specialist had been able to find this amazing liquid that completely wiped out the smell. It hadn't been covered by his insurance, so she had advocated [its purchase] for him somewhere, got the funds, and bought it for him. She had made it possible for us to be close again, to touch, to connect for the last time. I'll always be grateful for that. He died a few weeks later.

During the next phase of his education in AIDS caregiving, Danny began to understand the difference between "dying with AIDS" and "living with AIDS." In the late 1980s, many more people began coping with the long-term reality of AIDS in their lives. Medications were improving, care was improving, and people were changing their lifestyles, their nutritional habits, and their outlooks. Most of all, people began to resist the notion that an AIDS diagnosis was a death sentence.

During daily reports at the hospital, a doctor or nurse might make a prognosis that a particular patient wouldn't make it through the weekend. Afterward, I'd go to see the patient and I'd ask, "How do you feel? Do you feel as if death is near?" And the patient would say, "Are you kidding? I'm going on an RSVP cruise in March." Many times these same people who weren't going to make it through the weekend would walk out the front door of the hospital two weeks later.

These people say to themselves, "I'm not going to let this illness prevent me from going on my trip. They'll have to work it so I can carry my IV bag with me, because I'm going!" I've had many clients like that, and they're a real inspiration.

Once I expected someone would die over the weekend. Betty was in a coma. She was sixty-two, and had been an IV drug user for forty years. But when I came back on Monday, she was sitting up in bed and her sister, who had arrived Saturday, was braiding her hair. When the sister came into the room, Betty had come out of her coma. I saw miracles like that all the time.

The miracles Danny sees all the time contribute to his development as a caregiver, but they don't blind him to those less than inspirational moments, when you can only wish for a miracle to get you through. In those cases, in lieu of miracles, you may have to depend on your own judgment.

Danny had to make such a judgment call—in an environment that requires you not to judge your clients—while he was Shanti's residence coordinator:

The Shanti House is a model for independent living. We
don't go in and take over. But then Scott, one of our residents,
began acting psychotic. He had made a meal for himself and
ended up sleeping in it. His apartment was filthy, and he was
just a mess. But when I suggested that he go to the hospital,
he was very resistant.

I had this conversation with myself. Part of me said, "I
shouldn't be interfering. He has a right to sit in his messy
apartment." And yet I also noticed the cigarette burns on the
carpet, and I had to look at the larger picture: a building with
sixty-four people with AIDS living in it, and me insisting,
"He has the right to his independence," as the building goes
up in flames.

So then I asked myself, "What is your intention here?"
And my intention was that Scott go to the hospital and
get it together so that he could come back. Checking my
intentions reminded me that I cared about Scott; I wasn't
just trying to get him out of the building. And knowing I
cared about him let me tell him that he had to go into the
hospital.

I made the arrangements, and the doctors discovered
that it was a combination of medicines that had sent Scott
into a clinical delirium. While they were stabilizing him, we
had the maintenance people clean his apartment. When he
came home, he was fine.

Clearly there are no hard-and-fast rules for this kind of decision
making, but Danny demonstrates the difference between people-
managing and caregiving. Danny didn't know the right thing to do
for Scott. He had to look inside himself for the answer, and his way
of doing that was to ask himself about his intentions for Scott.
When Danny deemed these honorable—and he could because he
knew he *cared* for Scott—when he knew his decision would be
based on what he believed was best for Scott, he could allow himself to judge Scott's situation dangerous, and act. As it turned out,

what was in Scott's best interests was probably in the best interest
of Shanti House as well.

AIDS agencies that provide volunteer help to clients usually
designate one or more people as volunteer coordinators. Shanti has
four, and their roles are crucial to the success of Shanti Project.
They are the ones who match volunteers to clients; they are also the
ones who must decide whether the person who wants to take part in
the training to become a volunteer will be an asset to the project.

When I was a volunteer coordinator for Shanti, I interviewed
a woman for the training who I really didn't think was going
to work out. I had been describing how Shanti works, explain-
ing our peer counseling model, and so forth, and at the end
she looked very discouraged, and said, "But I came to Shanti
to give hope to people living with AIDS. I want to give hope."
    I told her that as a practical support volunteer, if she went
to someone's apartment and the bathroom was dirty and she
cleaned it, and that gave the person hope, that was one thing,
but that we don't send volunteers out with the intention of
giving hope. And I had to tell her I needed to hear that she
would be willing to abide by our policies and the way we
worked, because I could just picture her taking over someone's
life and deciding he needed to follow a certain path. But she
said, "Okay, I'm willing to do that."
    About three months later, her client phoned me, and as
soon as he mentioned her name, I had visions of her tying
him to a chair and hitting him over the head with a Bible.
But he said, "I want to tell you that this woman, she's very
quiet, she comes to my house, she cleans my house once a
week, but when she leaves there is this feeling of peace that's
in my house that you could cut with a knife. And this feeling
lingers there and it comforts me. And she doesn't say very
much at all."

It was wonderful. I told her about the call—she had really gotten it about how you can be an example by what you project—how you can give hope without telling [people] they need it.

Shanti clients have made many such calls over the years in praise of volunteers who provide invaluable service and do not preach to them. This is a fundamental aspect of the Shanti training model: volunteers do not offer advice about treatment, or promote their version of spirituality, or play therapist. Volunteers do offer practical, functional support, or peer support; they listen, they provide respect and validation, and as Danny demonstrates so well, they really *care*, which may be the most precious gift of all and for some recipients a first-ever experience.

ￋￋￋ

In many ways, human beings are very similar. When they have problems, it's often over their differences. As a gay, African-American man, Danny values what is different about himself as well as what is different about the people he meets, in and out of the job. One of the things he loves about San Francisco is its cultural diversity, which he told me "challenges white people to open up. But people of color aren't often challenged to be open to other cultures or races, which I've never understood."

Danny told me that he was prepared to encounter a certain amount of racism in his job as volunteer coordinator, just because he'd be dealing with the public. All sorts of people were calling, looking for help for themselves or for someone they cared for with AIDS.

I'd ask whether they'd like a man or a woman, and many times they'd respond, "Just don't send me a black volunteer. I don't want any blacks in my house."
Part of what allows me to handle racist remarks is because

I feel empowered as a black person. I can't say enough how important those early dance teachers were—their telling us how beautiful we were. They gave me an image of myself as powerful and proud. I still carry a lot of that.

Shanti teaches its volunteers that they will meet and work with all kinds of clients, some they won't agree with, some they won't even like. The point is to help the client. If Danny had told the caller who didn't want any blacks in his house that he was talking to a black staff person, he would not have helped the client, he would have alienated him—from Shanti, its services, and possibly other AIDS services.

But the reality is we often cling for dear life to our biases. We resist seeing through historical, prejudicial beliefs and attitudes associated with different groups— even though these have been dis- proven and should have been outgrown. Maybe we hold on to our prejudices because we don't have enough personal experience to revise them. Lacking meaningful contact with diverse groups, we have nothing to go on other than the old saws and stereotypical notions.

These may be so ingrained we aren't even aware of them. This is an area where consciousness raising is terribly important—to test whether our perceptions are based on facts or on biased preconcep- tions. Such a test is not confined to the standard gender biases or racial prejudices. Shanti trains its volunteers in "multicultural awareness." We ask, Do you have a judgment about eye contact? Did you know that in some cultures it is a sign of disrespect to look directly into another person's eyes? Do you reject illogical thinking? Might you judge someone by his or her style—assertive or low-key? And if so, why? We ask you to monitor how you respond to body language, conversational style, to people with physical disabilities. We ask you to remember when and where you learned your responses. Then you have to decide whether they are appropriate or useful now.

And when we find that we do hold prejudices, we don't condemn ourselves, we try to understand ourselves. We do this by bringing the dark thoughts into the light so we can examine them, and when necessary, modify them.

There's danger in reducing diverse groups into neat, easy categories. Talking about "women's needs," or "what to expect from Hispanic patients" only deepens stereotypes. Unless we're very careful, our efforts to train people in multicultural awareness could promote just the kind of stereotypical thinking it is meant to eliminate. But clearly, *ignoring* differences is not the answer, either. Culture, gender, race, sexual preference, education—all these, as well as one's personality and psychological functioning, interact to make the individual unique.

The solution seems to be what Danny has found to be so useful in his caregiving: to treat each individual as unique. As much as possible, to take the factors that contribute to one's individuality into consideration; to be aware of our similarities, and of any tendency toward bias, toward prejudice, or toward judgment when judgment is not called for.

We try to strike a balance between embracing the uniqueness of individuals and understanding the diverse backgrounds that people with AIDS and their caregivers are coming from. It's not a question of one or the other, but of one *and* the other: accommodating and respecting uniqueness and diversity at the same time.

3
Saying the Right Thing

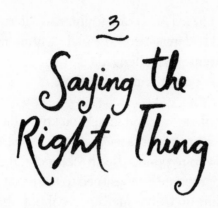

Cecilia Worth, R.N., one of the early promoters and teachers of the Lamaze method of childbirth in this country, is today a nurse at San Francisco General Hospital's Ward 5A. She had been living in New York in the early 1980s, working in obstetrics, when she read a newspaper story about a man who had died alone in his apartment, afraid to tell anyone he had AIDS. "I wept over the horror of it," she told me. "It really spoke to me. I have strong feelings about the rights of individuals to acceptance and respect, especially in times of trouble."

This stranger's story did more than speak to Cecilia. It shouted. And Cecilia did more than weep over it. She was fired to do something about it. She knew, perhaps intuitively, that to make some changes in the world she would have to start with changes in herself.

She turned from a devotion to life's beginning, to a focus on life's last stages for men and women with AIDS. She spent the next two years in New York as a home care nurse to people with AIDS, and in 1989 moved to California and took a two-month review of hospital nursing at Merritt Hospital in Oakland, California. That same year, she applied and was accepted at San Francisco General to work on Ward 5A. The work was intense. "Patient needs were far broader than I had imagined," she said. "My abilities to help and to learn were intensely challenged." For the next five years, her teachers would be her patients with AIDS.

> Somebody looks at you and says, "You know, I'm dying." There it is. Right in your face. You don't have the vaguest notion of how to respond. The checklist of ten things to say all seem inappropriate. I've learned to trust that my inner voice will come up with something, or if not, that it's okay to be silent. But I had to learn that. One person who taught me was Clyde.
>
> Clyde was a federal prisoner. He could hardly walk and he couldn't breathe without oxygen, yet he had two armed guards sitting outside his door. He was kind of chipper and jive. We got to be buddies, and one day he suddenly turned to me and said, "You know, I'm dying."
>
> I didn't know what to say: "Do you mean right now? Or just generally speaking?" Part of me wanted to run out of his room, but another part was all his. I sat down and put my arm around him, and we sat there without saying anything.

Clyde's lesson is an important one for caregivers. Precise answers may not be what a person is searching for when he or she reaches out with words that seem to require answering. Frequently, what's really wanted is a genuine expression of compassion, which can be a touch or a look when your heart is in it.

Cecilia listens to her intuition when she's at a loss for words. Sometimes it offers inspiration, as in the case of Jimmy:

> Jimmy was a gay, retarded man who had lived much of his life on the streets. His legs were so swollen they looked like tree trunks; he had an advanced pneumonia, extensive KS, and dementia on top of being so childlike. But he was very sweet. There was a tremendous innocence about him.

As he got worse, he began to call out fearfully that he was going to hell when he died. He'd say, "I've done some terrible things in my life, terrible things." I didn't know how to help. I couldn't say, "Jimmy, you're not going to hell. There's no such place." I asked myself what could he hear? And I thought of his friends. I said, "Jimmy, you know your friends Tim and Terry? They're really beautiful people, aren't they?"

He just glowed. His mask of fear disappeared, and he said, "Yes, yes, they are." And I said, "They love you tremendously, don't they?" And he said, "Yes, they really do, and I love them, too."

And I said, "Well, Jimmy, you know it takes one to know one. You love them because they're so beautiful. They love you because you're so beautiful." And he said, "Yes! That really is true!" "So just be aware of how beautiful you are," I told him, and for a moment he moved into a whole other perception of himself.

But then I'd leave the room, and two minutes later I'd hear him saying, "Oh my God, help me, I'm going to hell when I die."

I asked the rest of the staff to remind him how beautiful he was anytime he started talking about going to hell, and there were moments after that when he really experienced his own beauty. I don't know how he died, believing he was going to hell, or thinking he was totally beautiful. You can wish for things, but you don't always get them. At least he got moments of feeling totally loved.

Cecilia is especially sensitive to another person's fear. She acts intentionally in the face of it, "to bring in even a speck of space where the person can breathe, where they're not completely locked up in the fear." She borrowed on her experience with women in childbirth for this, soothing them through their labor, focusing with them on the contraction now, not the one just past or the one to come. Intuitively, she found something to soothe

Jimmy—his sense of his own beauty—and focused with him on that, not on what he had done in the past, nor on what the future might hold after death.

⸺⸺

The best caregivers try to be aware of the impact of their words on the ones they care for, but it's hard to foresee how grief or suffering, like interference on the phone line, may transform your words' reception. Sometimes you make a mistake and say something insensitive, or you say something innocent and it's taken the wrong way. Your words wound the one you want to heal. Then it's a gift to be able to say, "I'm sorry. That was a thoughtless thing I said." It takes humility to do so. But we are continuously humbled by the face of profound grief or suffering.

Sometimes you're surprised. You think you've said the wrong thing, when in fact, the opposite is true:

> A patient of mine had heard that I was one of the organizers of Lamaze in this country, and he had told me that he and his wife had used it for the births of their children.
>
> On this occasion, he had come in for a simple thing, the placing of a central line [a tube inserted in a vein for administering certain drugs]. But then complications arose—an infection and then a pneumothorax. He was already very weak and this tipped the balance. He was dying, and was unconscious.
>
> Several of his gay friends were there, and his ex-wife, very scared. When I came into his room she was sitting by the bed, and she turned to me and took my hand and said, "Thank you so much for all you're doing." And I said, "Geoff told me that the two of you used the Lamaze method. I used to teach Lamaze."
>
> Well, she absolutely collapsed. She burst into tears and

I thought, "Great, Cecilia, wrong thing to say." She held on to me, sobbing desperately, she couldn't stop. I thought I was going to stop breathing myself. I just stood there thinking, "What can you do for an encore?"

After maybe five minutes she finally got control and stopped crying. I squatted next to her chair and said, "I'm terribly sorry; that was a really dumb thing to say," and she said, "Oh no, not at all. It's just that there's so much we never said to one another. I thought he had forgotten."

I told her then how he had talked to me about what it had meant, sharing his daughters' birth, and how much they meant to him, and how he used Lamaze for his own pain and difficulty breathing.

It struck me that if he hadn't gotten the pneumothorax, his wife would never have been called, and if I hadn't said what seemed like a blunder, she would never have had any idea of how he held their relationship.

Caregivers are sometimes consumed by a fear of saying the wrong thing. Many search for a formula or model that will avoid their stumbling over difficult issues. Of course, it's important to try to be as sensitive as possible, but it's more important that the person with AIDS be allowed to express his or her feelings and be encouraged to talk about what's on his or her mind. It's not necessary that the caregiver respond "correctly," but that the caregiver listen actively and respond nonjudgmentally. When thinking back on a particular visit with a caregiver, an ill person will not recall precisely who said what, but he or she will remember that the caregiver was willing to listen.

Caregivers who focus largely on their client's or patient's problems and on saying the right thing run the risk of overlooking the person they're supposed to be caring for. It is often a great relief to novice caregivers to realize that they are not obliged to solve every problem or provide an answer to every challenge.

When I was very new on the job, I had a patient named Jack who was a tremendous manipulator. The first two days we were together, he had a dozen reasons why he didn't want to take his meds now, or have his bed made when I had the time to make it, or take some exercise when we had someone available for that. He would eventually do what I asked, but negotiating consumed a huge amount of my time and energy, and his stalling played havoc with my schedule.

On the third day, I walked in at 8 A.M. and asked Jack to take his pills so he could go down for an X-ray. Right away he started in again. And I snapped. I got this rush of anger, and I said, "Now listen, today we're not going to go through any of this stuff. You tell me yes or no, that's all. Yes or no, will you get up? Yes or no, you'll take the X-ray. None of this other stuff, is that clear?" And he said, "Got it."

Later that day he was up walking around, and I overheard him say to some buddies that he'd met on the unit, "My nurse really gave me shit today. That was cool."

That was very interesting to me. It was a lesson in setting limits. A year later I got a telephone call at the nursing station from Jack. He said, "I just wanted to tell you I never forgot you."

If Cecilia had given Jack her ultimatum on her first morning with him, she probably wouldn't have had the same result. She gained his respect and cooperation only after she tried to accommodate him for two days. He had seen her sincerely try to meet him halfway, and when she'd had enough, he saw the sincerity of her insistence that he quit messing around.

Cecilia, for her part, had taken the time to "see" Jack, to acknowledge his wants, to consider his position. "Being seen," as Cecilia puts it, is crucial to healing because it validates the individual. Delia's story is a poignant demonstration of how some people must fight for that validation:

> Delia was a black woman in her thirties, very poor, very downtrodden. She had come in with PCP so severe that she had to be intubated. Intubation is meant to get someone over the hump, not to be a way of life, so after she had been in the ICU for two weeks and was still alive, the decision was made to take her off the respirator. There was a chance she wouldn't make it, but Delia survived. In fact, she got stronger, and was soon returned to our unit, although without a voice. The tube had damaged her vocal cords.
>
> The second day I was with her, she was sitting up, and beginning to walk. It seemed like a miracle. But then she began to be restless, and when I checked her oxygen saturation I saw it was going down. I put on some more oxygen, called the docs, got an X-ray. She had had a spontaneous pneumothorax. It's always such a blow. Especially with severe PCP, your lungs get so fragile.
>
> Her intern came in, and said, "You have a hole in your lung, Delia, so we want to put a tube in there through your chest." And Delia shook her head, she didn't want it.
>
> The doctor's attitude was, "Delia's a street person, no education, what does she know?" And she explained it again to Delia in a patronizing sort of way. Delia shook her hands and her head no. The doctor looked nonplused and got the resident, who explained about the air building up outside the lung that would soon cause it to collapse and would eventually put so much pressure on her heart and the other lung that she would die. And Delia said no.
>
> The next doctor who came in offered to make it a small tube, and the next doctor suggested, "We could do it with a needle, we could just pull out that air . . ." Delia just looked at them. Someone finally went for the head honcho, and he

asked her if she understood that she would die without the intervention, and she nodded yes. And then they made her repeat the words, and in this very careful whisper, mostly just mouthing the words, she said, "I understand that if I don't get the tube I will die and that is acceptable to me."

Everyone stood there, in awe of her. No one was scornful or thought Delia was ignorant any more. Her resident told her that we admired her and respected her decision and would do everything to make her comfortable.

After everyone left, I explained that if she experienced any pain, or when she began to feel short of breath, which she would, that she could have morphine, which would help her relax and eventually fall asleep, and that she would die in her sleep. And Delia nodded, almost imperceptibly, that she understood. She was asleep before I left, but I did get the chance to say, "Delia, it's been an honor to be with you." Delia took her own power. And she died that night.

What Cecilia calls Delia's "power" in this circumstance, her knowing her mind, and insisting on acknowledgment, and getting it, was very moving to Cecilia. "In the midst of the incredibly unfortunate reversal of her life expectancy was her triumph of being seen and heard. I was struck by how peaceful she was."

Cecilia, like other of our caregivers, speaks the language of the wounded healer. "When someone else is seen," she observed, "it relieves my pain." Her own early sense of herself helps her resonate with those others who are "unseen," passed over as insignificant, who aren't listened to, or who are ignored or disbelieved. In early childhood she herself had been raised by disinterested domestic help, and felt unseen and unheard. Frequent household moves disrupted friendships and childhood security. When she told her parents that the longtime gardener had molested her, she was spanked. When a city inspector took her down into the basement and abused her, she went to her mother again, and was told not to tell lies.

Cecilia's isolation as a child, her inability to elicit comfort or support or even acknowledgment from her parents in her worst moments allows her to identify at some primal level with Delia's circumstances. That identification motivates Cecilia to support Delia's "taking her power," as well.

* * *

Florence Nightingale, who helped revolutionize nurses' training in the mid-nineteenth century, observed that the role of the nurse is to build a healthy environment for patients to heal themselves. In large measure, this refers to the human environment, the relationship between patient and caregiver. Any relationship takes time to build, and time is what hospital nurses have in very short supply.

On 5A you are supremely busy, physically, mentally, and emotionally, every second of every day. You have to know an enormous amount in terms of caretaking, medications, technology. Your priorities can change every minute. You have to be able to move fast. The demands are incredible. People say, "We had this wonderful nurse." They have no idea. Being a good nurse, which includes offering practical and emotional support, challenges everything you've got.

Cecilia recalled her patient, Clyde, the prisoner on the ward who had said, "You know, I'm dying." "At exactly that moment a doctor walked by whom I had been trying to reach, I heard myself being paged, and someone had just told me that the patient next door had lost control of his bowels." The hospital situation allows little time to be reflective, for processing what's happening, for personal growth, or for commiseration. When Cecilia sat down with Clyde and put her arm around him, even for that minute, she demonstrated her renegade style of nursing.

Physicians and nurses and other caregivers have a powerful impact on the patient, and a powerful influence on the patient's attitude toward his or her illness and its treatment. A great deal of what caregivers communicate is expressed nonverbally, through their tone of voice, eye contact or lack of it, and body language. In the hospital so much of the nonverbal message is, "I'm busy. Please, no heart-to-hearts right now!"

Such an unintended, unspoken message can be demeaning and frightening to patients who have already surrendered themselves to their doctors and nurses and hospital routines, and are asking only for reassurance. In fact, the whole system of surrendering oneself to the medical team in charge runs counter to the kind of healing environment Cecilia and many others would prefer to offer, one that fosters restoration and strengthening of the self, not the surrender of the self by either patient or caregiver.

I watch people fall through the cracks. Somebody is labeled a "difficult patient" and some of the staff start mentally bypassing them, looking at the illness instead of the patient, as if they're not really there. It makes me furious.

In such a challenging hospital environment, caregivers like Cecilia are often the last connection with a seriously ill person's humanity and his or her inner resources. It is a privileged position from which a healer can help an individual access the psychological and spiritual strength to survive. I include "spiritual strength" because I mean more by survival than physically making it through another day. My definition includes that *and* a search for inner peace to settle some of the unfinished business of a lifetime.

But how does a dedicated nurse go from writing a few words in a patient's chart about his or her "psychological status" to becoming a person who can offer real emotional support? Continuing education workshops and crash courses in the psychiatric or psychosocial aspects of AIDS care are only the beginning. Mastering the art of psychosocial care requires serious self-inquiry, an education in key areas of psychology and psychiatry, and most of all a willingness to let the client be the teacher. Such a reversal of roles may seem revolutionary and unsettling, even frightening at first.

For opening ourselves to our clients' or patients' humanity means reckoning with our own feelings of grief, fear, and anger. At the same time, our vulnerability is also the source of our empathy and compassion, the keys to the best kind of caregiving.

⟍ ⟍ ⟍ ⟍

Like other wounded healers described in these pages, Cecilia's approach to caregiving has to do with "connecting your pain with their pain."

The problem is in knowing what to do with the pain once you've opened to it. Suffering is hard on everybody. It can build up and overwhelm you. I struggle with that. My biggest challenge is to figure out how to be joyful and peaceful while being open to the suffering.

What Cecilia says reminds us that nurses and other caregivers who spend countless hours supporting people in a life and death struggle need support themselves. Hospitals rarely have time for adequate emotional support of their patients, nor do many support their staff caregivers, the nurses and other health care professionals who work there. And where support groups do exist among hospital caregivers, they are hardly encouraged, and frequently poorly attended. Cecilia tried to maintain one for the staff on 5A, but it was eventually canceled for lack of attendance.

The notion that emotional and psychosocial support is optional, or worse, unnecessary for professionals will spawn a reality that treats only diseases and not people, and that will undermine caregivers' effectiveness and the well-being of the ones they serve.

Too often our efforts to remain efficient are born of the notion that being emotionally accessible to our patients (and to ourselves) means compromising rational judgment, and/or sacrificing time management. But Cecilia believes that it is just as important to hold someone's hand and listen deeply to what he or she is saying as it is to check oxygen levels and give medications on time. She believes that her patients possess inner resources and strengths that can be drawn on to meet the challenges of healing, and she trusts her own inner resources to help patients find theirs.

4

I Show Up, I Pay Attention, and I Care

Usually, when I walk into a hospital room at 5A, I pray, "Help me do the right thing."

There's a lot of surrender involved. I have to step out of the way, and it's scary. Sometimes things I do don't work, or they don't seem to work, and then I have to sit with my own inadequacy. It's hard to feel inadequate. But that's life sometimes.

Micaela Salort is one of the most respected caregivers in San Francisco, a model for the field, who embodies the concept of the wounded healer: her history helps her to connect with and care for people who are suffering, and that connection and care comes back to her, replenishes her, and renews her.

Micaela moved to San Francisco in 1978 at the age of twenty-one. Her initiation into AIDS caregiving occurred several years later, when she and other lesbians began ministering to their gay male friends who were "getting sick really fast with incredibly strange symptoms."

Some of these men I had considered co-parenting with, and they were getting sick and dying. It was very frightening. And of course, my ideas of having a child went out the window.

We set up a rotation of friends to visit them, because when they're sick and home alone, you know that they're not eating, or they need help to go to the doctor. So we had shifts, and we kept in daily contact by phone.

That the gay and lesbian community would rally round their stricken friends seemed natural to Micaela:

Where I grew up, my godmother lived down the street, my godmother's sister was across from our apartment house, my grandmother's best friend was on the same block. If my grandmother wasn't home when I got home from school, I'd go to any one of those houses and be welcomed like one of the family.

If anybody became sick or needed something, the community was there. You depended on it. For me, there was more a sense of security in the community than at home.

Her community was Spanish Harlem. One of Mica's early memories is of going to Puerto Rico with her grandmother to visit her great-grandparents when she was five years old. She recalls her great-grandmother "hallucinating and talking craziness," the product of syphilitic dementia, she thinks now. Her great-grandfather was blind from syphilis. The old lady referred to Micaela by her mother's name, which was terribly disconcerting to the little girl.

But this was not Micaela's first experience with craziness. She recalled her bipolar (manic-depressive) paternal grandfather; her frequently depressed grandmother; an alcoholic father who played sexual games with her and her brother at bath time; and a mother driven to pull herself and her family up and out of their tenement apartment.

Mica's mother accomplished this by working full time and attending school at night. She finally did earn a graduate degree and get a mortgage on a small tract house in the Bronx when Micaela was twelve years old.

The four adults in my life were very damaged people. My mother was one of the darkest skinned in her family, which made her the brunt of a lot of racist stuff—aside from which, she hadn't been well cared for by her own mother. My father grew up in Hell's Kitchen in New York, was orphaned when he was a child, and saw a lot of horrors in World War II—he was one of the liberators at Dachau—not that he ever talked about any of that to us. My grandfather's mania demonstrated itself in terrible rages against my grandmother.

Somehow, I became the family counselor. From the age of four, I sat there and listened to it all and tried to make peace and tried to make everyone feel better.

A child who bears the weight of her whole family's ills usually does so hoping that her responsiveness and nurturance will be rewarded in kind. Deprived of the loving care of those people who matter most, as Micaela was, we will trade almost anything to win some of what we so desire—even our childhood.

Mica worked hard to please her parents and grandparents, to be the glue that held the family together. But her caregiving service to them was self-sacrificing—she sacrificed what she felt and wanted and needed—and self-depleting, because she got back none of the nurturance that she put out. What she has learned in the years since is still about sacrifice, as she gives of herself, but it is a kind of transformative sacrifice, which fulfills Micaela, rather than depletes her.

As her own family's counselor from a very early age, Micaela picked up some skills that have become second nature to her, and clearly contribute to her talent as a caregiver. She learned vigilance, for one thing. And she is equally attentive today, as I've had the opportunity to observe in the experienced caregivers group we both belong to. I watch Mica watching—she's very good at it. She watches to see who's okay. She does it very gracefully; she's never solicitous or overbearing.

I have the sense that in a way, not much has changed. Micaela's focus has always been the wounded other. She seems to me to be the grown-up version of that young observer and counselor who was—and is—valiantly there for those who need her. But her evolution from self-sacrificing caregiver to one who gives of herself without giving herself away, means that everything has changed.

〜〜〜

Micaela's change began when, in spite of her sacrifices, she was still not successful in gaining the loving kindness and attention she craved from her sadly dysfunctional family. In her teenage years she found refuge elsewhere—at the Cloisters monastery in New York, in alcohol and drugs, with the Moonies, and then in psychotherapy and dedicated self-scrutiny, and finally in the Hindu ashram that is her long-term spiritual home.

Her inner work, the passage of time, her loving nature, and her devotion gradually began to heal the damage that her lost childhood had caused her. Micaela came to define herself—the Micaela under the caregiving mantle, the essential Micaela—as someone with feelings and needs and desires. This shift in self-definition changed her work with clients fundamentally—from self-sacrificing caregiving to transformative caregiving.

> I've done a lot of work. I'm thirty-six years old, and most of my adult life has been about trying to heal the damage of my childhood. Once, when I was about fourteen, I was really sick. I had a 104-degree fever. I was hallucinating. No one cared. And this was not unusual for my home environment. My brother and I weren't cared for until we collapsed, passed out, and had to be taken to the hospital.

There was tremendous denial and an inability to see suffering and be able to deal with it in my household, and I think about that when I'm with someone who's living with AIDS.

I know that my efforts to provide some love or healing touch or words to my clients are also my efforts to heal the child in me who was not taken care of at home. But taking care of someone else *does* heal me. If I'm able to heal another person or help another person heal, it's a circular thing. It works for both of us.

This reciprocity is at the heart of the wounded healer's relationship with the wounded partner, and it generates the highest moments in caregiving. Micaela demonstrates this in a story she tells about a man named Jonah:

Jonah had been out on the street all his life. Talk about suffering—he was a junkie, he was a dealer, he was a mess. He had legs the size of tree trunks from the KS, he was demented, he was gone. But he was very, very sweet.

I was passing his room and saw him out of the corner of my eye trying to get up out of bed on these very unstable legs. I ran in and caught him just before he fell. I got him back into bed before I understood he wanted to go to the commode, so I helped him do that, and then put him back to bed again. It was clear he wanted to talk to me, but I couldn't understand a thing he said.

I don't know whether this was because he was demented, or because his teeth were like floating in his mouth. You know, there's that terrible gum disease that comes with AIDS sometimes, where the teeth are just floating in your mouth. [This is periodontitis aggravated by AIDS.] So I really couldn't understand a word, but I was there. I sat on his bed, and it was one of those moments of surrender where you just go for the heart, and I started praying, Please, I don't know what he's saying. And I tried very hard to listen to him.

And then after several minutes, he looked at me clear as day, and he said, "Baby, I don't know what you're doing, but whatever it is, it's working." And then he just lapsed right back into noodle time.

It was like the sun shining through the clouds. It's a moment in time. But I was very touched and very moved by that moment, and I know he was too. For that moment he wasn't a crazy junkie dying of AIDS, and I wasn't Micaela with all my history and who I am. We were just timeless beings in a crystal clear moment. And then, of course, he lapsed back into being a junkie dying of AIDS, and I was me again.

The transcendent moment that Micaela describes, when the ego melts into the background and the boundaries blur between oneself and another, is a spiritual gift. Such crystal clear moments illuminate Micaela's spiritual path, and bathe her own pain and humiliation and neglect as a child in their restorative light.

Many caregivers come to the spiritual life as a *result* of their work, searching for a transcendent purpose for the suffering they see; but some, like Mica, come to the work as an *expression* of the spiritual life. She told me, "I was always searching for God and meaning. I went from devout Catholicism to Eastern philosophies to Transcendental Meditation to the Moonies to where I am now. I always wanted to know the truth and to serve the truth."

✐ ✐ ✐

In 1987, when Micaela took a job in Information and Referral with Shanti Project, both she and Shanti had been caring for people with AIDS for about the same length of time. From 1989 to 1991, Micaela worked for the Center for Disease Control in New York as a field researcher studying gay men at risk for HIV. Part of this job trained her in pre- and post-HIV counseling. When she returned to San Francisco, she came back to Shanti and for three years worked as a counselor at San Francisco General Hospital's Ward 5A. When I asked what she did there, she responded, "I show up, I pay attention, and I care." Until recently, Micaela was Shanti's training coordinator, imparting her expertise as a caregiver to hundreds of new volunteers.

The kind of care she provided as a peer counselor, however, is the subject of this chapter, and that was exceptional. She has a talent, learned from the practice she had with her family, to assess need as well as to address it. I have seen Micaela in action. She has a kind of thoughtfulness that comes from her intentional focus on her work, what she calls "being present." She counts on that "presence" to tell her what to do when she isn't sure what the right thing is.

You walk into a room and you're faced with a myriad of possibilities, and anything can happen, and has happened. Every family drama is played out in these rooms. Unspoken things are spoken, hurts and anger held for decades are let loose.

I remember once at S.F. General finding this drunk, hysterical woman sitting on the floor next to her husband's bed. He lay paralyzed with AIDS complications, and she was screaming, "Daddy, don't leave me!"

The nurse wanted to call security, but I asked him to let me see what I could do. I sat down on the floor next to the woman and put my arm around her and said, "This really sucks, doesn't it?" And she went on screaming, "Daddy, don't leave!"

Then I said, "You know, maybe he wants to know how much you love him. Why don't you get up on the bed with him and put your arms around him."

And I helped her up and she lay down with him and held him, and I left them that way.

This is the voice of the archetypal wounded healer who hears the pain of another as her own. Micaela embraces the opportunity to make a deep connection with one in need. She calls it her "practice," and speaks of it in spiritual terms: "My practice is trying to experience the eternal connection with another person." She uses her intuition for this, and her education, and physical touch:

> I find that one of the most important things I can give someone is a loving touch, because in the hospital they're constantly prodded and poked and hurt, and all the touching they receive is about pain.
>
> I had a patient named Richard, in his fifties, an accountant. He was having his first bout of PCP. His lover of twenty-five years had died the year before, and all his other friends were dead, except for a woman who was his next-door neighbor. He loved good food, he loved to cook, and he had an incredible music collection, which he had given to the San Francisco Conservatory of Music. As he got sicker, he said listening didn't thrill him any more.
>
> I knew it was his last hospitalization—he was going to be transferred to the hospice at Laguna Honda Hospital. As a goodbye gift I told him I wanted to give him a massage, and he said, "Wonderful."
>
> What I didn't tell him was that I had a ninety-minute Maria Callas cassette with me. I had told the nurse what I was going to do so she wouldn't bother us. I put the tape on quietly, and began the massage. The room was dim, and as I was stroking Richard's feet, the room filled with Maria Callas—just to think about it gives me goosebumps.
>
> He opened his eyes and stared at the ceiling, and then his eyes filled with tears. I was silent, I just kept touching him. After her aria, he said, "I had forgotten how beautiful." That's all he said, and then he just sobbed, and I held him. It was our last time together. He died a week later.

Micaela's caregiving is no longer offered as a bargaining chip for affection and regard. It is an expression of genuine love. It says to all those she serves, to Richard, to the grieving wife of a dying man, "I choose to be with you in a healing partnership. I will stand with you in the midst of despair." The statement represents Micaela's spiritual commitment.

She attributes her ability to live and work in the moment, to be joyous and spontaneous, to experience another's pain and sorrow, to be creative and playful, in part to her spiritual commitment, which includes early morning devotions at the ashram. This is the place where she can "be quiet and not even think about anything."

But she knows that a spiritual commitment alone is not sufficient to heal past wounds. Her commitment to her psychological development is as strong as to her spiritual growth.

I had a therapist friend who told me that as long as you keep trying to solve all your psychological problems through spiritual means—by meditation or prayer or by assuming the solutions lie with a force greater than yourself—you're really avoiding dealing with your problems. I didn't believe it at first, but now I think it's true. When I realized avoidance was not going to work—because the pain was still going to be there—I had to start facing some pretty hard things.

For one thing, she faced her past. Micaela had sat and listened to everyone in her family but herself. She had tried to make peace for everyone, but had none for herself. She made a conscious decision to do so now. She gave up alcohol and drugs. She "decided to think a great deal." She went into therapy, and not just one kind of therapy, but Jungian therapy, transactional analysis, radical feminist therapy, and reevaluation co-counseling. She danced with the Sufis.

What she learned was that to deny her pain was to hold on to it. It was only when she was willing to go through it, feel it, name it, talk about it aloud, that she could learn from it and be relieved of it. It was then possible to find joy, to know spontaneity, to be in the moment, to feel another's pain and sorrow, to open to creativity and play.

▰ ▰ ▰

In 1986 Micaela broke her ties with her mother.

I had cabled my mother a dozen roses for her birthday, with
a card that I'd signed in this cutesy way, "Much love on your
birthday from your firstborn." Cost me fifty dollars. She never
responded, and much later I asked her if she ever got them,
and she said, "What roses? Oh, those! I thought your brother
sent them." To her, her firstborn was her firstborn son.

I had been giving my ear, my understanding, my heart,
my patience, my reflecting back to her whenever she called
up to complain about her life—my healing presence, all my
life. I was tired. I had tried so hard to please her, to be the
A student at Bronx Science; I even went to medical school
for her, though I didn't want to and dropped out after a year.
And for her, basically, I didn't even exist.

Her mother's demonstration of disregard registered with Micaela
like the last straw. It was then she stopped sacrificing herself to
another's manipulation and became her own guardian. From then
on, mutuality would characterize all her caregiving relationships,
and the perpetual feeling of being shortchanged, exhausted, and
often angry would fade. It was the beginning of Micaela's transformation from one who gives without self-renewal and is therefore
always on the edge of depletion and despair, to one whose giving is
regenerative and reciprocated.

It's interesting that the work doesn't debilitate or exhaust
me. Stuff around it, all the bullshit trappings and political
garbage at the agency or at the hospital exhaust me. Co-
workers who don't pull their weight exhaust me. But I feel
rejuvenated after two hours with a patient who is being real
about the nightmare he or she is living.

This is not a paradox in the world of AIDS, and certainly not in Micaela's world, where her spiritual life is pervasive and paramount. It frames her perspective and sense of priorities.

You know, I consider that the other person is a manifestation of God in a particularly intense reality that won't go on forever. It won't. And death may come as a welcome release. For some people, approaching death is the opportunity to go beyond this reality, to get to a higher place. For some it's not. I try to remain steady and nonjudgmental whatever the process. Suffering is going to continue, and people will get sick and die and have to face a lot of stuff.

Caregiving is heart work. But it's not easy work. You experience some hard things, some ugly things. It's hard to help clean somebody up who's soiled himself for the fifth time in a row, and do it with love, and do it so his dignity remains intact. But if I can bring my love there for them I think it helps them, heals them, transforms them; and I've been with enough people while they were dying that this has been validated for me.

━ ━ ━ ━

Now Micaela gives her ear, her understanding, her heart, her patience, her reflection, her healing presence reciprocally, not as a unilateral sacrifice. She is replenished by moments of success, by small progresses. And she experiences special joy in the toughest cases. "They test who we are," she told me. Mark was considered a particularly difficult patient:

He insulted everyone, threw things at people, yelled and carried on. I had been avoiding Mark. Everybody had. But then someone stole his cigarettes, and he went nuts. Mark had no one in the world. His cigarettes meant a lot.

I bought a pack of cigarettes, took a couple out of the pack and slipped them into a little bag with some chocolates that were being passed around the ward. Then I went to visit him. I said, "I heard somebody stole your cigarettes. I'm really sorry. Here, have some of these," and I left.

The next day I went by his room again, and again the next day, and sometimes I'd just bring him chocolate, and sometimes I'd include a couple of cigarettes.

Then one day as I passed his room, he yelled at me, "Come here, come here, sit down, look at this!" It was the AIDS Quilt on TV—one of the soaps was using it in an episode. Mark and I watched it together in silence, and then he began to cry hysterically and to tell me about his lover whom he had made a panel for, and all this pain and anger poured out, and I sat there and listened to all of it turn to grief, lots and lots of grief. And after that day it wasn't as if he let go of his anger with everybody else; he was still difficult, but something transformational had happened, and he let me be with him when he was dying.

Micaela considers these especially challenging cases "central to my path and my transformation. If I'm just going to deal with patients who like me or think I'm great or who are easy to deal with, that's not going to do it."

I actually love going to the Psych Ward, where a lot of counselors won't go because it's just too much for them. But my clinical training began when I was four years old and fielding my grandfather's bipolar mania. So when I saw a man admitted with a bipolar diagnosis, I went to see him. He was pacing in a tight circle. I introduced myself to him, and he said, "I need to pace." I answered, "Can I pace with you?" and he said, "No, I need to pace alone." I said, "Fine, but if you ever want someone to pace with, you know where I am. Just call me."

The next place I saw him was on 5A where I was working. He didn't want anyone in his room, didn't want to talk to anyone. He had open, suppurating herpes zoster all over his body, and his nurses were finding it hard to touch him. So I offered to give him a massage. Of course, I wore gloves, but it was still very difficult.

I remembered something that my friend Bharat uses to help him through the hard places. He repeats to himself "This is my guru in a distressing disguise." I made my mantra, "This is the guru massaging the guru. This is the guru massaging the guru."

Our whole relationship transcended. It was amazing. I'm massaging this man, and out of nowhere he says to me, "Have you ever had creme fraiche?" And I said I had, and he said, "What's it like?" And soon we were talking about how he wished he were in a sidewalk cafe in Paris.

After the massage he asked me to come back soon, and I did, and then it was just about sitting with him and reading to him. And this was the man who had gone from pacing on the Psych Ward to a fetal position on the AIDS ward, to creme fraiche. Miracles can happen.

✂ ✂ ✂

Micaela's clients speak in superlatives about the love she lavishes on them. In some respects, caregiving is all about love—"heart work," as Micaela calls it—and she is a passionate lover.

I sincerely believe that the lover is more blessed than the beloved. The love I give comes from me, and the love I feel is mine. Somewhere deep inside there, in spite of all the pain and hurt and all those scars, there's that endless well of love.

That endless well of love exists in all of us. It is central to our humanity. But sometimes circumstances or family or other influences obstruct our access to it. Finding our way through the obstacles is hardly ever easy. Micaela is threading her way with psychotherapy and spiritual work. Because it means so much to her, she has arranged her life to keep the accessway open to her inner life. Her spiritual devotion supports that goal. Her "practice" of connecting to the eternal in another person sustains it. Her commitment to "be present," to pay attention, and to care, manifests it.

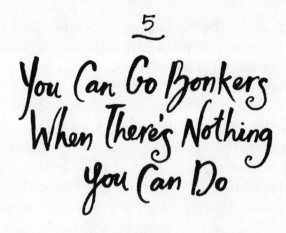

5
You Can Go Bonkers When There's Nothing you Can Do

I was supposed to die first. I was diagnosed six years ago.
My brother was diagnosed six months ago. He was a nurse.
He was supposed to take care of me. That was the way it
was supposed to be.

Larry Hjort was diagnosed with AIDS in 1986, and, believing that
knowledge is power, immediately turned his considerable intellect
to the task of learning everything he could about the disease.
Because the discovery of the virus is relatively new, it has been possible for dedicated individuals to follow the growing medical and
scientific literature. (In San Francisco, moreover, it has been possible to comprehend much about the disease by attending to one's
friends.) Many people with AIDS have made the effort. It is a way
of gaining some semblance of control over the capricious and often
terrifying turns AIDS may take.

In another effort to take charge and shore up the personal
resources he knew he would need to live with his disease, Larry
went into therapy. He considered becoming a volunteer for Shanti,
but "was afraid that it would be too difficult for me. Too mirroring

of my own fears." In 1989, however, he decided to confront his fears and take the Shanti training. To this day he is glad he did—and not just because it prepared him for the then-unanticipated care of his brother.

> I knew it was going to be difficult because I was also sick.
> I was afraid that being Chris's caregiver would drain me.
> I had a hard time working out a boundary for what I could and couldn't do for him. Toward the end, I lost my boundaries.
>   Chris started having complications much more quickly than I had. He'd get sick on and off, and then he started losing his mind, and things changed overnight. Then somebody had to be with him all the time, because he was mobile, and he had all these plans, and he'd walk out the front door and simply disappear. You had to catch him to stop him.
>   I had to take his keys away from him, and his checkbook, and it was very painful for him because those were symbols of his independence.
>   He shifted in and out of dementia, and sometimes he knew when he was rambling and in a different world, and he'd come back for a bit. And there I was, telling him where he was at: "Okay, Chris, here's what you just said—here's what it sounds like." Finally he asked me to stop being so honest because it hurt him.

Larry's experience with his brother was a stark lesson in how none of us succeeds in caregiving all the time. Chris didn't appreciate Larry's feedback on his dementia, and loving concern on Larry's part appeared to Chris like restrictions of his freedom. Larry's deep desire to help had collided with the conflicting reality that there was nothing he could do about the way the disease progressed in his brother, and, as Larry put it, "You can go bonkers when there's nothing you can do."

> The "fix-it" part of me went crazy. When you love somebody

a lot and you're watching this deterioration, you want so badly to do something. It's enough to kill you, but you can't do anything. You have to tell yourself, "There is nothing I can do but be here. I can't change this. I can't make this better." You have to know how to take care of yourself so that it doesn't drive you crazy enough to jump off a bridge or something.

The situation caused Larry a great deal of pain, but even during the worst of it, he was aware that he had to accept his limitations as his brother's caregiver, or forfeit his effectiveness as a caregiver altogether.

As it turned out, the lessons got tougher.

The night before he died, Chris was very agitated because it took so long to administer his medication. He was still upset when I said goodnight and went upstairs to my apartment, which was right above his.

Tuesday morning when I went to see how he was doing, I found him on the outside back stairway. He was still alive, but cold as ice. It was January. It was about fifty degrees outside. He had locked himself out of his apartment—the door must have slammed shut behind him—and my door was locked. I don't know how long he had been there.

A neighbor helped me get him into the car, and I took him to the emergency room. The doctor there was a friend of mine, so that was good. We talked about Chris's chances, but they weren't good, and soon it was apparent that Chris wasn't coming back. He was too weak. I don't think he wanted to come back.

So he died in the emergency room on Tuesday morning. It took me weeks to calm down. Your mind goes crazy with, "If I had only done this, if I had only done that. If we'd rearranged this, if we'd made these plans, none of this would have happened."

But I finally realized that I could do that until I drove myself bonkers, and I still would not have any answers. The "what ifs" will never be answered in my lifetime, and to keep asking them is self-flagellation of the highest order.

Central to our understanding of limits, and our potential as caregivers, are such questions as, What can I actually *do* for the people with AIDS whom I care for? Can I undo my brother's suffering? Can I eliminate my client's grief over the losses he or she is experiencing? Can I compensate this friend for the lack of love in her life? for bad breaks? for socioeconomic disadvantages? Can anyone remove the hurdles that exist for another person?

Larry had to answer for himself how much physical help to offer Chris, and how much to encourage his self-care; whether or not to take his keys away; how to respond to his growing dementia; how to motivate him, lift his spirits, ease his pain. AIDS makes the answers to these questions especially difficult because the patient's needs and capacities may fluctuate dramatically from day to day. It is not unusual for caregivers to be afraid of misjudging, of making a terrible mistake, and many believe that they do not do enough, and some conclude that they were not adequate to the task. Larry had to put aside his guilt.

> I've come to terms with Chris's death. I don't know what put him on the back porch, but something did, and in the end, because he was so unhappy about the dementia, I think he saw being caught outside as "This is my opportunity. This is my window." He could have gotten back in if he had made enough noise. He was capable of doing that, but he didn't. So I have to believe it was his choice.

〟〟〟〟

The Shanti *training* had allowed Larry to accept the whole concept of caregiving, when he was thinking in terms of his own eventual needs: "[Before the training] I would have been resistant to caregivers around me. I would have been conflicted about need-ing care, wanting it, and hating it." What the Shanti *volunteer work* taught him was all about boundaries—that place between too remote or inaccessible, and too identified with the client.

One way of maintaining the boundaries is by clearly defining the caregiving role you intend to fill. A caregiver may be a friend, a nonjudgmental companion, a sounding board, an active listener, a counselor. A caregiver may interact with health professionals as an advocate or coordinator of his client's health care. A caregiver may pay bills, go shopping, manage household chores and the client's personal business; he may dispense medication, help with bathing, arrange social activities like visits and outings, keep his client's friends and loved ones informed of the client's status; he may help the client manage the symptoms associated with HIV disease and its opportunistic infections.

The caregiver's role often changes over time as the relationship with the client matures and as the client's needs change. This may extend the limits of the caregiving relationship; but even then it is not unusual for caregivers to establish firm limits and stick to them—for example, not performing certain aspects of personal care. The caregiver's commitment to the client in such a case would be to find other assistance to negotiate these tasks for the client if he or she required it.

Effective limit setting allows the dedicated caregiver to estab-lish a healthy interplay between self-sacrifice and respect for his or her own needs. It is interesting that when caregivers learn to con-sider their own needs legitimate and respond to them attentively, they are able to meet their client's needs more fully.

Too often, enthusiastic caregivers start out trying to be best friends with their clients, and wind up leaving caregiving work in less than a year, disillusioned and drained. Often they have underesti-mated the responsibilities and the commitment caregiving requires, or the time it takes to build a close, trusting relationship. Then they must reassess their commitment and their boundaries, and the time they are willing to spend on the caregiving relationship.

The lesson about boundaries has been one of the most important in my life, if not the most important. Without the training I would have gotten far too involved with my clients. I would have been too emotionally bound up.

I don't think it comes naturally for a person to say, "Wow, there are an awful lot of things here I can't fix and I can't control, and I have to just be with that." I think it's our nature to try to do both. Reading that we can't fix it or control it isn't going to change our nature. The real knowing comes in experiencing not being able to help, experiencing your limitations.

You have to feel your inadequacies deeply enough to get it that, in fact, there is nothing to do. It's hard because we're accustomed to thinking that we can do something about our illnesses—that a shot or some pills will make things better. When they don't get better, you have to find peace with that.

The lesson here is that there isn't such a thing as inadequacy in these situations. Inadequacy is a human invention, it's a judgment we make. It doesn't really exist. In fact, everyone is perfectly adequate. There are just some impossible situations.

Although most caregivers acknowledge that certainly there are limits to what one can do, many have great difficulty accepting this and making it operational in their own lives. They're confusing limitations with inadequacy, and inadequacy suggests blame or guilt. Even Larry uses the words interchangeably. But Larry knows, better than most, that not being able to do for someone has little to do with personal inadequacy.

The caregiver who accepts his limitations—and here the word is *not* pejorative, only what's real—is a caregiver who doesn't try to control or fix everything for his client, and isn't besieged by guilt over his inability to make any big changes, and isn't driven to do more than his personal limitations allow.

And as much as we hate to admit it, there are some people we simply cannot help, some people with whom we are not well suited for partnership, some clients with whom we can never establish a caregiving relationship no matter how hard we try. Honesty and humility in these situations is at the heart of caregiver wisdom.

Even the wounded healer, who crosses from the world of illness to the world of health, must acknowledge the boundaries between the worlds. When caregivers are reluctant to draw a boundary between themselves and the people they care for, when they identify too completely with the client, when they insist on being responsible for and sharing everything—when the caregiver and the receiver merge, in other words—they risk not only failure, but harm.

Establishing boundaries and keeping them was especially hard in Larry's caring for Chris. How could he not identify with his beloved brother? And because Larry had AIDS too, how could he not project himself into Chris's battle with the disease?

Two things saved Larry: his intuitive understanding that there were inviolate boundaries and real limits to what he could do for Chris, and his abiding love for his brother. Larry had answered for himself the question of how much he had to offer Chris, even if he sometimes ignored what he knew about his limitations. His boundaries may have slipped with his brother, but the perimeters held.

It was because we had certain bonds. We loved each other unconditionally. It was that simple.

That's the reward in the work—being in that state of love. I've finally gotten that. Unconditional love expects nothing and has no conditions. It feels wonderful. I dance for joy when I'm there. Of course you don't go around, "Gee, I was in unconditional love today," or most people don't. But that's what this is all about. And unconditional love takes some of the pain away from the fact that people are going to die.

For me it has been very difficult to get to where I feel secure offering unconditional love, that I'm not fearful of being hurt by loving that way. Several days ago I hung a sign on my kitchen cabinet: "It's unconditional, stupid," just to remind me.

✐ ✐ ✐

Larry is a frequent speaker at my class for first-year medical students at the University of California Medical Center. He talks eloquently about the patient/doctor relationship—our TV-inspired assumptions of it, and the truth of it. At its best, it is an intimate relationship, maybe especially intimate when the disease is AIDS; and it shares some of the same emotional range and content of other intimate relationships, from love to hate, from anger to equanimity.

I'm hard on my doctors because I want them to be partners, resources, equals. My doctor may know a lot more than I do about medicine, and I give him credit for that. But he doesn't live in my body. I want a person who hears me and consults with me instead of dictating to me, who acknowledges that I may not know as much as he or she, but gives me credit for what I do know. Ultimately, I have to make the decisions, and a lot of physicians don't see that.

I asked Larry what happens when his doctors don't acknowledge their partnership. How does he educate them?

As opposed to merely firing them—which is what I've done in the past—I stand up and say, "You're not listening to me, you're not paying attention, you're not giving me credit, and this isn't going to work if you don't."

I understand they need to keep their boundaries clearly defined or they would be drained dry by now, but imagine you're the patient: you've been lying on a cold steel table in front of the CAT scan for an hour and a quarter with a six-inch-long needle in your liver. The physician is digging around trying to get the perfect biopsy sample and your

morphine is wearing off. He keeps saying, "Just one more
section, just one more sample." His impatience shows when
you say, "Not without some more painkiller." You have to
fight with him for another 15 minutes before he haughtily
agrees.

Physicians are caregivers—or should be. I want one
who's present, preferably one with empathy, who knows who
I am and cares about me.

Larry likes to refer to himself as "the patient from hell." His personal physician for several years has been Tom Schiller, whose story also appears in this book. "He listens to me," Larry tells me. "I have a great deal of respect for him. We may yell and scream at each other but we work it out."

When Larry discusses his relationship with his physician, he's clearly talking about a collaboration in which he and his doctor have equal status. Yet Larry knows that his own contribution to the partnership is likely to lessen as his energy wanes. Calculating the patient's limits in the caregiving partnership is therefore a dynamic process. Caregivers and patients must periodically adjust their expectations of one another based on the physical, psychological, and emotional state of the person with AIDS, and sometimes on the changing life situation of the caregiver.

✔ ✔ ✔

Unless caregivers are clear about boundaries as they relate to their clients, about how close for how long they are willing to get, and what they are willing and not willing to do, they run the real risk of losing their effectiveness in the relationship. One way this occurs is when the caregiver allows his or her own problems to cross into the territory of the partner with AIDS.

As a patient going through my own issues, I've learned that
I don't need—I don't want somebody encumbering the situa-

tion with his unresolved emotional stuff. And as a caregiver
I try to be conscious of not putting my issues out there so that
my client doesn't have additional things to deal with.

As a person with AIDS and an experienced caregiver, Larry's
perspective on the disease he lives and works with makes him especially sensitive to the expectations a person with AIDS and his or
her caregiver have of one another. He can help people with AIDS
sort out the emotions that threaten to overwhelm them; he can
help caregivers recognize the boundaries that keep them effective.
He says, "I have an idea of what caregiving should look like—of
what I want it to look like." That idea has evolved through Larry's
volunteer work as a peer counselor for Shanti, through his experience with Chris, and more recently through his work as a support
group facilitator for long-term survivors of AIDS.

Out of all that experience, he has also concluded what caregiving *doesn't* look like; and as he works to stay conscious of not adding
to his clients' burdens, so he tries not to be oversolicitous, and not
dismissive:

I saw this with my brother and a friend who was visiting.
Chris began to get up to get something, and the friend was
right on top of him: "Here, let me help you, let me get it for
you." But Chris didn't need help, didn't ask for help, didn't
want help, and he snapped at his friend to leave him alone:
"Don't do that, I'm fine, I'm capable of doing this, and I'd
rather do it myself."

But nothing frustrates me more than to mention some
physical problem I'm having and have the other person
attribute it to something perfectly benign. For instance, I
get anemic and I tire very easily. If I were to say that I had
a hard time walking up the hill today, and you responded,
"Oh, it's just because you're getting older . . ." well, that's
very frustrating.

Of course, a person says something like that to soften what you've just said, but it doesn't acknowledge the truth or the reality of the situation, and it drives everybody I know with AIDS nuts.

Larry's vision of what caregiving should look like also incorporates an understanding of control as an issue for both the person with AIDS and the caregiver. And this is much more complex an issue than who's in charge, as Larry made clear with this graphic explanation:

Think of someone whose world is shrunk down to the table at the side of his bed. All the control he has left is over that table, and he exercises it by moving things on the table, arranging things a certain way. Then to have someone come in and thoughtlessly move the table or be unconscious as to the importance of how things are placed on it—it's very painful.

Caregivers in such situations need to be aware of and respect their clients' diminishing control over diminishing worlds. This is another aspect of respecting another person's boundaries.

6

Sometimes My Feet Go Numb

Sometimes my feet go numb
I sleep a lot
Most of my old fag buddies are dead
My doctor treated my lover too
I feel guilty about being alive.

Sometimes my feet go numb
In people of color the skin is ashy dry
Coffee and tea don't go well with my medication
I remember sexual freedom.

Sometimes my feet go numb
It takes one to two days to get a prescription filled
   at San Francisco General.
I heard two guys making a speed deal at the Food bank once
My thumb nails are blue from AZT
Bruises that don't heal quickly worry me.

Sometimes my feet go numb
My sweat smells medicinal, my urine stinks
Television commercials make me cry
The news makes me angry
I'm tired all the time.

Sometimes my feet go numb
I take an anti-depressant and other drugs
  to scare my voices away
I hate pity
The very idea of wearing diapers is humiliating
I wonder if the acupuncture is doing any good.

Sometimes my feet go numb
And I don't notice until I try to walk
Then I stumble
  swear
Shake them awake
  and move on.

Wayne Corbitt is a poet, a playwright, and a man with AIDS who became a caregiver when David, his lover and companion, got sick with AIDS in 1986. David died two years later. Wayne described their relationship.

We had made a lifelong commitment to one another. We used to say we were going to be two old queens in Stinson Beach lusting after the boys together.

The week he died, the only thing he would eat was melon. This was in February, so I had people running all over the place to get him honeydews, cantaloupe, and watermelon. When he died, I was holding his hand and singing "You Are My Sunshine" in his ear.

He had always been the one who took care of me. He was sort of the man of the house. But as he got sicker the roles began to reverse. Then he started having psychotic episodes and I was really forced to take over, which is something I never thought I could do. I was always so needy, and suddenly I had to be there for him.

How did you do that—make that transformation in yourself?

Well, in a way, living with and knowing David had sort of prepared me for it. I grew up a sissy. I was a sissy boy. I didn't have many friends and people made fun of me. I got beat up a lot and pushed around a lot and the only safe place for me was to hide in my room when I was at home. When I moved in with David, that wasn't tolerated. Hiding wasn't allowed.

David believed in me when I didn't believe in myself. He believed I could do things. He always said that I would be a famous poet. Well, I'm not famous, but I'm a poet that some people know. And I've had some accomplishments— I've had a play produced, which I didn't think I could ever do. And people ask me to do readings. I'm not going after any of this stuff. It all comes to me out of his predictions and his faith in me. He really believed in me.

David's belief in him enhanced Wayne's self-esteem. Wayne began to see himself through David's eyes, and that became a source for the personal strength Wayne needed to become the provider for his lover and partner. But it also made the idea of David's dying especially painful. What was he going to do without David standing in the back of the hall during his poetry readings, loving and supporting him? Wayne thought that his personal strength might rely on his lover's reinforcement. Without David, he feared he might revert to a kind of frightened passivity, or worse.

I'd be making dinner and David would yell in to me about something ordinary and all of a sudden I thought of him not being there. I felt pure terror.

One of the last times David went in the hospital I went into crisis because I thought I was losing him. To be very honest, I thought I might crack up.

When I asked Wayne how he kept from cracking up, he attributed his sanity during these hardest times to his friends:

I was very lucky in that I had friends who helped me out with David. In the beginning when I could leave him alone, I sometimes went out to a bar, or dancing. But then when I couldn't, I had to ask for help. So I'd call my friends and say, "I need to get out of the house," and someone would come over for a couple of hours.

It's really important to do that, to get out, to just forget about it and not feel guilty; otherwise it festers. You get pissed off and resentful.

The leather community also offered Wayne a system of support and a source of understanding. AIDS has hit this particular community hard, and the survivors are especially sympathetic to the effects of the disease. Wayne told me:

I had friends who were into leather and the South of Market scene. They helped. There was a sex club that I used to go to called the Beat Boot Camp, where they had a "Monday Night Opera Society." It was slow on Mondays, so they played opera on the video. We talked dirty and drank beer. It was a real relief for me.

Leather men are always so butch and tough and everything, but they cry easier than anybody in the world and they're more sensitive to what's going on with AIDS. The leather community was a real important support system for me. Because they're all freaks to begin with and there's nothing you can do to shock them. Crying isn't shocking at all.

And I was crying in those days. At the time I was working at a restaurant on 24th Street with this prima donna chef who was very screwy, and at home David was having these psychotic episodes, so he was very screwy, and sometimes I would sit out back at the restaurant and smoke a cigarette and want to run away from everything. There were times I really didn't feel like coming home.

Finally, I called Shanti for help. They put me together

with a very nice man whom I saw for the next seven months or so. I saw him for about five months after David died.

If you're taking care of somebody, you have to take care of yourself. If you think you can do it all, you're fooling yourself. But one of the hardest things for me was to say, "Okay, we need an attendant here. Okay, I need some help." David and I cried, we cried a lot.

✎ ✎ ✎

The strength to survive comes in many forms. Wayne had support on a community level from friends; he saw a Shanti volunteer for those seven months as a way of taking care of his psyche; he had a creative outlet in poetry that gave him an arena for soulful exploration and expression. But learning how to take care of a loved one with AIDS is often accomplished "on the job." Wayne talks about some of the routines he and David worked out:

David and I slept together, and it became a routine that he would wake up covered with sweat, and I'd push him over onto a towel and lay a couple of clean towels down, and he'd roll back over next to me. It was the least fuss. Or he'd say, "I've got to go now," and I'd help him up on his knees and stick the bed pan under him and he'd do his number.

Boom, boom, boom. This is what we do with night sweats. This is what we do when he has to shit. This is what happens when he throws up. And because we got into such a compartmentalized routine, we were able to enjoy life, if that makes sense. We rented movies, we played Scrabble. I cooked for him, and he always ate well—high protein and low fat, no oil, no red meat, but a lot of herbs. Cooking for people with AIDS, you keep it very simple.

There came a point where he couldn't go out of the house without some help, so I did that, and then he became incontinent, and so I changed diapers.

Wayne reminds us that when people with AIDS become more and more ill, loved ones, friends, and volunteers may have to take on tasks they're not familiar with. Caregiving may require giving injections, cleaning wounds, and changing diapers. Health professionals and community agencies may offer classes or workshops so that caregivers can learn these skills and not feel overwhelmed by new responsibilities. Still, there can be times when it all seems too much to bear.

> We had a rule. You have two hours to feel sorry for yourself. More than that, I can't handle. I just couldn't. It applied to me too.

It was a good rule. Setting limits is another survival necessity that takes on-the-job training and isn't as easy as it sounds. You can deceive yourself into thinking you're doing just fine, while your stress level mounts as grief intensifies inside you. And even when you recognize that you do need a break or must set some limits, you may have to search for the courage to say so.

> It's a hard thing to do because the person you're saying it to is sick and dying and deserves sympathy and empathy and help, but you have to draw a line somewhere and say, I'm not going there.

David became more difficult as his disease progressed. People suffering with some forms of mental deterioration may demonstrate the kind of rage that David experienced with increasing frequency at the end of his life. Anger is one of the few emotions powerful enough to ward off terror. It makes the person who experiences it feel a resurgence of strength. It comes with a little adrenalin; one's muscles contract to it. It's active. It feels vital. But for the caregiver/witness it can be excruciating.

> One time we went to the hospital for a transfusion for David. These transfusions make you feel great for a while, and David

really needed to feel good. But when we got to the hospital, [SFGH's outpatient] Ward 86 was pandemonium. There were people lining the hallways, the waiting room was full to overflowing, all the beds were taken. It was just awful.

David had to lie down, and I badgered a nurse into giving us a bed in the back of the examination room. When I told him, David threw a fit. He screamed at me, "I want a real hospital room, not this! I want to be checked into the hospital, and I don't want this shit!"

He was carrying on, ranting and furious. I had to tell him, "You can't do this. I'm trying, the nurse is trying, we're all trying. This is the best we can do until a room opens up, and you just have to be quiet." After that I got him settled and walked away and broke down.

Treating him like a petulant child was the hardest part. Telling him, "You can't do that," and "I won't tolerate this." It was especially hard because David had been so competent. He was very smart, educated in philosophy and theology and religion. He was deconstructing and reconstructing before it was fashionable. He had a brilliant mind, and suddenly it wasn't there in the same way. It freaked me out.

◢◢◢◢

Wayne has moved from a position of learned helplessness where he felt at the mercy of life's circumstances, to a place where he experiences an enduring feeling of effectiveness, and increasingly, his own competence and talent. Wayne is no longer merely a spectator of events around him. Now he is a participant and contributor.

To a significant degree, Wayne's contribution has been his art, which is nationally recognized as among the best depicting how it is to live and love in the era of AIDS. For us, it is a portal to understanding some of his world in these times. For Wayne, it is a means of self-expression that helps stabilize him psychologically and nourish him spiritually. He told me:

My T-cells have been less than 100 for five years, and at
one point they couldn't find any! I can still walk around.
I get tired really easy, but I'm still here, and one of the reasons
I believe I'm still here is my writing. I believe that God blessed
me with this gift. If I didn't have it, I wouldn't be here doing
all this stuff: readings, play being produced, visibility nationally. Still, on occasion all this so-called success rings a little
hollow.

Why?

Because the people I would most like to share it with aren't
here. I've lost fifty-five friends since 1984. Every time something really good happens, the sadness creeps in that they
aren't around to see it. Especially those who didn't think
I was going to amount to anything. Especially them!

━ ━ ━ ━

To some of us, Wayne looks like a hero. But his heroism, like
that of other caregivers and people with AIDS, is not based on the
old notion of dying for a glorious cause or ideal; it is based on life
affirmation. By continually summoning the courage to survive in a
world suffused by death, by responding to the extraordinary challenges of everyday life with AIDS, Wayne and his colleagues uphold
the value of life and of the human spirit. It was in this spirit, after
David died, that Wayne decided it was "payback time."

When David was sick we got a lot of help from the hospice
and from visiting nurses. David was real personable, so all
these people loved him and really took care of him. After
he died and my T-cell count dropped to where I couldn't
work as a line cook any more, I decided it was the right time
to pay back some of the kindness.
    I chose Shanti. But during the training program, I didn't
think I could do it. But when David got sick I didn't think

I could do that, either. I was afraid because being HIV positive, I knew I would be coming face to face with my own future.

During the volunteer work, I had four clients. The first one was a white man who was a speed freak. I had been a speed freak at one time, and I couldn't handle this guy's using. I didn't want to be around him.

The next three were all black men who were very close to death. Alfred was one of them, sixty-five years old, bisexual. One was Mark. One was Orlando. I watched these kind black men, these incredibly beautiful people, be sick and die. It made me less afraid. There are a lot worse things than death.

- - - -

As a man with AIDS who has cared for men with AIDS, and now receives the care, Wayne can speak about caregiving with a special passion. He has redefined himself in the course of his caregiving experience. He had believed himself a weakling and victim. He has become a competent, gifted survivor. He has discovered from his supportive friends and from his clients that survival is a collaborative process. Surely his survival is also linked, as his effectiveness as a caregiver most certainly is, with his willingness to keep learning about himself and to let his self-image change with his new knowledge.

But self-knowledge is difficult and fraught with denial, and change frequently meets with resistance. It requires ever-increasing trust in our intuition and intelligence, and continuing faith that we can do what needs to be done, to persevere in the world of AIDS. And probably as important as increasing trust and continuing faith for the caregiver is that we acknowledge our humanness, that we recognize our fear, anger, grief, resentment, or despair, and that we find healthy ways to express the thoughts and emotions that arise with these reactions.

So we must find someone to talk with, someone who will listen;

we must give ourselves permission to cry and rage. It's only when we've cleared a path through this heavy emotional terrain that we can begin to think creatively and to make constructive choices in response to our own changing needs and those of the people we care for.

7
How Did You get AIDS?

I tell women who are going into the hospital, never admit
how you got AIDS. Always say, "I'm not sure." If you don't
want to lie, tell the truth: you probably don't know whether
you got it from IV drug use or unsafe sex, so you're not sure.

Mary Corwin is an articulate advocate for people with AIDS. She
has been living with the disease herself for more than ten years, and
has been in and out of hospitals for drug and AIDS-related problems. She knows the ropes, both from inside drug addiction, and
from outside—she's been clean for nine years. Mary is much in
demand as a speaker at conferences on AIDS. Her advice about not
divulging how one contracted HIV is based on experience and
observation.

My daughter, Sinead, once asked me why I never told the
nurses how I got it. I said, "I'll show you." The next nurse
that walked in, I said, "I think I probably got it from my ex-
husband," and she was just all over me with sympathy and
let-me-fluff-your-pillows. The nurse who came in after that,

I said "I got it from IV drug use." She was in and out of that room in five minutes flat. Sinead and I were hysterical laughing. That's how open the prejudice is.

It's the same with doctors. Their attitude is that a female with AIDS got it through unsafe sex, which is unfortunate but not the end of the world; or she's a victim—she got it through blood transfusion, in which case she's like Mother Teresa; or she's an IV drug addict or a whore. In that case you did it to yourself, you get no sympathy, and the care you get will reflect which category they put you in.

Health care professionals who operate, consciously or not, out of the premise that "junkies and whores" with AIDS "deserve it" may act out this discriminatory belief in the form of reduced attentiveness to patient needs—although they will likely deny this. If the caregiver believes that all IV drug users are manipulative and conniving, then he or she will approach such people as adversaries. The caregiving relationship will be a kind of contest that the caregiver wants to win.

Some caregivers know that IV drug users are more often disenfranchised street people who have been alienated and abused by the system, and are understandably, if not justifiably, at odds with authority. Still, their patients may be operating on the assumption that the doctor doesn't like them and is likely to give them less than the best care, and so they try to connive for better treatment—and the prophecy is fulfilled. The more each side argues over who is to blame for the difficult relationship, the more each validates that it *is* someone's fault. This creates an atmosphere of right/wrong, suspicion, and mistrust.

Our perception of reality is shaped by our direct experiences as well as by our beliefs. It seems to me that we not only believe because we experience, but we experience because we believe. It takes a lot of honest self-scrutiny for caregivers and patients to acknowledge that what they thought was "reality" was strongly colored by their points of view.

Mary demonstrates with a personal story how appearances may influence another's perception of reality:

> I had walked into the hospital—barely walked in—with
> pain in my lower right side that was so severe I couldn't stand
> up. I couldn't talk. It was the most intense pain I've ever felt.
> I had been into the emergency room before with different
> stuff, and the ER physician and I had never gotten along,
> ever. For some reason, from day one, we just banged heads.
> On this occasion he told me to get out of his waiting room,
> that I was in there scamming for drugs and he didn't have
> time for it.
>
> I was too sick to fight. I was five years clean at the time,
> but I was dressed all in black with my leather jacket and
> boots. If I had come in with a pair of penny loafers I'd have
> been in bed in half an hour. Instead I left with my friend
> Carla and we drove around until that doctor's shift was over,
> and then went back. They checked me in right away with
> kidney stones.

Many health professionals who work with people with AIDS have been educated in the traditional medical model in which it is in the patient's best interest to be open and above board with the doctors. Doctors and nurses and other caregivers want to believe that their patients are telling them the truth. They may be uncomfortable working with patients who they believe are trying to trick them—"scam them for drugs," as the doctor said to Mary. After dozens of incidents of being manipulated by drug users, a cynical attitude is not so strange. But after treating IV drug users with AIDS over time, many caregivers soften with the understanding of how difficult the lives of many of these patients have been. Caregivers should be aware, however, that compassion is a response rarely trusted by many members of the IV drug culture, who may view such attention or intervention with suspicion. It takes consistency and patience to overcome their doubts.

✂ ✂ ✂

Mary was a child of a middle-class East Coast family who began doing drugs when she was twelve years old. She got hooked on heroin "in a relatively short time," she told me. "It doesn't take much to turn someone into a junkie, especially if you're shooting drugs to cover some deep kind of pain." Mary quit after twenty years, but by then she had acquired HIV. In her appearance in Peter Adair's critically acclaimed PBS documentary, *Absolutely Positive*, she tells us outright that she got it "by putting a rig into her arm." Many of her friends, drug users like herself, had been infected that way, too. Most had no family, and many went without treatment. Mary became a caregiver, as many of the caregivers in this book did, by caring for her friends.

When my friends started getting sick in the late 1970s, early 1980s, there was nobody there for them, period. AIDS was considered a gay disease. It wasn't being dealt with outside of that community.

Besides, traditionally, IV drug addicts don't look for care, and wouldn't follow through with it even if they found it because the care was never compassionate; it always revolved around them using [drugs], not around the fact that they were sick. A lot of these people were single parents who weren't able to access services because there was nothing in place for their children. You can't bring children to [SFGH's out-patient] Ward 86 for five hours while you wait for your appointment. If the kids don't kill somebody, somebody will kill them.

Then the best thing you could do for someone was to take her children while she went to the doctor. That's the kind of void that existed in the beginning. And we filled it, friends helping friends.

When AIDS first made its presence felt there were no formal

volunteer resources available. A friend would show up at a sick friend's apartment with a pot of chicken soup, and she'd notice that the house needed cleaning or the laundry had to be done, and she'd do it. When Mary discovered that she was infected with HIV, "that put a whole new twist on it for me. There were no services, no family, no one to really care, no one to fight for me. I began to get active out of rage over the injustice of it." Mary felt that rage for herself and for the others like herself whom she was caring for. She told me, "We were a family more than just a group of people. I mean, who wants fifty members of your family who are all drug addicts, but that's who I was with and that's who they were."

As the gay community organized around the disease and became more active, providing volunteer support, community services, and counseling, Mary noticed that women were consistently being left out—especially women with children. Her observations began to shape her caregiving and the kind of support she directed toward others.

My role became more and more to stand with people, to be one person who understood what they were going through, someone who would advocate for them, because of the intense hostility you got at a hospital once you were identified as a drug addict. To get decent care from that point on was a battle, and nobody can fight when they're sick. But one of the things that keeps me alive is to fight.

One quality that characterizes many long-term survivors of AIDS, like Mary, is their fierce determination to live. They demonstrate this by challenging their doctor's decisions, by asking a lot of questions, by bringing outside information to their doctor's attention. It doesn't help to relate to them as "difficult patients"; they're not trying to assert their rights or play a power game with their caregivers. Survivors like Mary are trying, day by day, to stay alive. When they themselves are caregivers, they bring their ferocity to bear for the best care of their friends or clients. Mary says, "It was natural for me to go with my friends, to make sure that they weren't put in a bed next to somebody with TB, to make sure that they received the same care as anybody else. There was nobody to do that for them. It's changing now, but ten years ago that's the way it was."

A lot of these people who came to S.F. General were also part of the methadone clinic, so I'd have to coordinate their getting their methadone while they were in the hospital. I got a lot of resistance. The doctor would say this isn't an immediate concern, we can put this off for a day or so, and I'd say, no, it is an immediate concern, and she's going to be really sick in an hour, never mind tomorrow, and then she won't stay—she'll leave the hospital.

Another problem was someone entering the hospital in pain and not being given pain medication because of her addiction, as if to say that addicts have less pain, or their pain isn't as severe as someone else's. Actually it may be as severe, but for your medication to be effective, you're probably going to have to give the addict a higher dose than you'd give someone else.

Also, it was really hard to get nurses to answer their pages. Drug addict patients were considered a pain in the neck. If you were advocating for that kind of person, you could sit there all day long asking when is her sheet going to be changed? You've changed everybody else's, now let's change hers. A lot of this stuff was done by friends.

Caregivers must remain aware of how strongly our feelings and beliefs about authority figures, IV drug users, women, gays, doctors, and so forth, influence our experiences and our behavior. As caregivers our effectiveness can be strongly affected by our judgments, moral or otherwise, about the lives or behaviors of our patients, our clients, or our colleagues.

Unfortunately, not all caregivers understand and adhere to this principle. It seems clear that a person with AIDS who is also a drug user should have a friend or relative who can be his or her advocate at the hospital, preferably one who is not easily intimidated and isn't afraid to make a fuss and to ask difficult questions. By and large, the more interest the advocate shows in the patient's care and health, the better hospital care that patient gets.

Mary is that kind of interested caregiver, and because she knows the culture and language of the streets, she is often an interpreter, as well. She tells Carol's story as an example.

Carol was a real street girl who had no idea how to deal with authority. All she knows about authority is lockdown. It's the streets or jail; that's her revolving door. I heard that she had gone stoned to the emergency room for something AIDS-related, so I went down there, and the doctor was screaming at her, and Carol wasn't responding to her questions. They needed to know exactly how much dope she'd had so they'd give her the right amount of drug for her AIDS problem.

I think doctors, when they deal with drug addicts, start with the presumption that this is someone with almost no I.Q. And I think there's a tendency, if you don't get the answer you want, to raise your voice more and more so that you intimidate the person into an answer. This doctor didn't know that if you're a drug addict and you've been living most of your life on the street, screaming is just a form of talking. You don't hear it as a threat. Carol probably thought, she's saying something but she's saying it too loud, and so what? But this doctor was going to put this girl into a narcotic withdrawal because she wasn't getting the answers she wanted, and that's wielding a lot of power.

I went in and I shook Carol's shoulder, and she opened her eyes. I told her, "They need to know what drugs you did so they can give you more or less medication." And she said, "I did a speedball, I did this, I did that." And I said to the doctor, "Do you have any more questions?"

◢◢◢

Aside from her commitment to her friends and to herself, Mary has another powerful incentive to stay strong—her fourteen-year-old daughter, Sinead. The two are exceptionally close. Sinead is aware of her mother's illness and the implications of it, but Mary still tries to shield her from worry. It's harder to insulate herself from worry, for even organizations that help women with AIDS don't usually provide necessary services for·their children.

Mary told me about visiting a major AIDS service organization in San Francisco that works specifically with families. She met with the head of the program there for women and children and said that she wanted to arrange a guardianship for Sinead, "and this woman looked at me and said, 'How do you do a guardianship?' "

Clearly, this is a major problem in the world of AIDS caregiving. It means that one of the biggest issues for women with AIDS who have children is not being adequately addressed. And this is not the only deficiency in a system of care that was conceived to assist a gay middle-class male population. Such a model simply doesn't work for children or for the needs of poor or disenfranchised women. On the most basic level, even medical services are hard to come by for these women.

Assuming you don't have your own private doctor, getting any kind of decent care from a clinic, getting any kind of gynecological care, is impossible. Until maybe three years ago [in San Francisco] there was only one gynecological clinic a month, that was it. And that had to be fought for. Finding doctors who are even willing to deal with women who have AIDS is really difficult.

Some effort is being made to fulfill other needs of women with AIDS, however. Shanti's volunteer support for the family members of people with AIDS is one movement in that direction. Jennifer Akfiret has been Sinead's Shanti volunteer for the past five years.

Mary and I talked about some of the implications for her vis-à-vis Jennifer's caregiving. Her comments are as thoughtful and honest as she is:

Mothers are supposed to be their children's responsible party, their providers. Mothers are supposed to feed their kids, clothe them, and send them off to school. When you take us out of that role and somebody else steps in to fill it there's a natural amount of resentment and hurt, even though we know this person is here to help us, not surpass us.

Mary is right: the parent-child relationship is not a partnership of equals. Parents normally care for children, not the reverse. Even older children, like Sinead, may not be emotionally able to be a parent's caregiver; and some parents, like Mary, find it hard to accept care. When she does accept it, she does so as much for her daughter as for herself.

I don't like to go into the hospital until the wheels fall off, but I had another bout with kidney stones and I was really concerned because it was just me and Sinead living together; there was nobody else at the time. Jennifer had come over and she said to me, "You don't look so good," and I whispered back, "I don't feel good." I didn't want Sinead to know. And Jennifer turned to Sinead and said, "Why don't we do a sleepover at my house" and she organized everything. About a half-hour after Sinead was out of the house, I was in the hospital. Jennifer's caregiving is to take care of Sinead so I can go to the hospital without worrying about her.

It's easy to see that a big part of helping Mary is assisting in whatever allows her to remain a nurturing, supportive mother for Sinead. To Mary, and to many mothers like her, no other issue in the struggle with AIDS comes close to this in importance. But even the most expert caregiving on Jennifer's part can not eradicate Mary's concerns for her daughter. She admits that she worries about Sinead.

> I don't want to see her heart broken. She's already gone through it so many other times—friends dying of AIDS, Carla, Billy, Tommy, James. That's a lot of death for a kid to walk through by the time she's fourteen. I'm afraid it will harden her.
>
> But when I try to talk about my passing, she's like, "Oh, God," and walks into her room. She's in therapy, and I think they do talk about it there.

In addition to their children's well-being, parents want their children's respect. They don't want to appear vulnerable, as they may when they're sick—as they may when society scorns them for having engaged in unsafe sex or IV drug use and gotten AIDS. Many parents try to hide the origins of their disease from their children as well as from their physicians, fearful that their children will make the same judgments that society has, and reject them.

In general, telling the truth works out best. Mary believes that the reason Sinead handles the fact that her mother has AIDS as well as she does "is because we've always been honest with each other about what's going on. She's never hidden my diagnosis from her friends and she's had no bad experiences. Maybe it's because no one in our extended family hides it."

The truth may elicit sad feelings, guilty feelings, regrets, and these may complicate honesty with our children, but not talking about obvious issues only exacerbates a child's fears. Children fear abandonment. Some who try to tough out rough times may not ask difficult questions, even though they have them. The most difficult question of all, of course, is, what will happen to me? Whether a parent with AIDS approaches this decision gradually or outright, it's vital that she let her children know who will take care of them after her death.[1]

The children of a parent with AIDS are often fearful that the parent isn't caring for herself well enough. They worry about her health and about all the other things the parent is normally responsible for: food, rent, bills. They may begin to see themselves as their parent's caregiver; they try to assume the role of an adult.

Children may not express their worries directly. They may act them out instead, becoming unusually depressed, or withdrawn, or aggressive. Parents or caregivers who observe this kind of change in a child can encourage the child to express his or her concerns directly. Mental health professionals who deal specifically with families or children can also help, although experience has taught some single parents with AIDS not to risk it. There is a pervasive fear of losing one's children to Social Services.

It hasn't happened to me, but I've seen it happen to friends of mine, where the mother goes into the hospital and suddenly Social Services is there asking, "Are you too incapacitated to take care of your children?"

Well, what standard of incapacitation do we use? If you've just been in the hospital, you'll probably be in bed for another two weeks. Is that incapacitated? Who's doing the cooking? The fourteen-year-old. This is nothing new to poor people in America; this is how you get by. But when you add a disease to the formula, you're on very shaky legal grounds.

It's one thing to be single and be able to languish in the hospital for two weeks until your symptoms have cleared up. For a woman with kids, you're in and out of there as quick as you can be because you're afraid that if you stay too long in the hospital, Social Services is going to take them away.

The fear of separation is a terrible additional burden for a mother with AIDS and her children. Especially in these cases, AIDS is a family affair. There's no question that the family that deals with AIDS together goes through some rough times, whether the family consists of a single mother and child, or a partnership, gay or straight, or parents and children. But Mary says, "People shouldn't die in the hands of people who don't love them."

There doesn't seem to be any question, either, that people living with AIDS gain some of the strength to survive when they are surrounded by people who love them and want to share the burden of the disease.

At the very beginning of the epidemic, when it was still called GRID, I knew a woman named Sally with maybe eight kids. She didn't have children, she had a tribe, all under the age of twelve, one or two still in diapers. She was a single mom, living on welfare in the projects back East. She had two rooms, no heat. It was the dead of winter.

I used to spend the night with her and as many kids as could fit in one bed—not just because there were only two small beds, but because you could keep warm that way.

These kids totally adored her. She never raised her hand to them, never raised her voice. And they took care of her. There were no social services then, or we didn't know about them. I made the food and they all fed her. Watching the way they were with her, it was like watching angels. And the sicker she got, the more tender they were with her. They bathed her and dressed her and took turns going to school so someone was always home with her. It taught me not to underestimate kids, especially their power of healing and love. She lasted a long time because of them, and not in total misery. I think there are a lot of kids who are willing to love people like that.

Sinead is one of those kids. And when Mary remembers how Sally lasted a long time because of her children, we know that she is also thinking about her own long-term survival because of her own beloved child.

Note

1. In deciding what sort of legal arrangement to make between children and surrogate parents, it's important to seek advice. There are three options: custody, which designates someone's temporary responsibility for the child; guardianship, which assigns certain, but not all parental rights; or adoption, the legal equivalent of biological parenthood. California is also one of three states that has the option of co-guardianship.

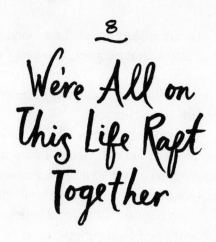

8

We're All on This Life Raft Together

I first saw a female doctor on "The Doctors" when I was five years old watching soap operas with my grandmother. I remember telling my grandmother that I wanted to be a doctor, and she said, "You mean a nurse." I said, "No, I want to be a doctor." From then on every year for my birthday she made me a white doctor's coat. It was this incredibly affirming gesture that said, "That's what you want to do? That's fine."

Lisa Capaldini entered medical school in San Francisco in 1978, around the same time that AIDS, by most estimates, began its deadly stalking of that city's streets. By 1983 when she graduated, San Francisco was recognized as an epicenter of the disease, and San Francisco General Hospital, where Lisa did her residency training, was a national model for how to cope with the crisis.

Her first choice after finishing her residency was to stay on at San Francisco General, but there were no openings at the time. Instead she joined two other doctors who had set up a clinic in the city's Castro district, primarily for gay men with sexually transmitted diseases. Within two years both her clinic partners had died, one of AIDS, the other of a heart attack. Lisa found herself running the private practice alone. In retrospect, Lisa says, "Having chosen to come to medical school here, and having done my residency at San Francisco General Hospital, and having landed in this clinic, there's almost a feeling of destiny to it."

San Francisco is fortunate to have had Lisa's destiny in its future. Unlike too many of her colleagues, Lisa is not just an intimate stranger engaging in routinized and impersonal treatments of patients. She incorporates a compassionate dialogue between her patient and herself into her caregiving, and believes that this is as crucial to the patient's self-healing potential as trust between patient and doctor.

The field of psychoneuroimmunology, or PNI, where researchers study the interactions between or among mental states, behavior, the nervous system, and the immune system, may bear this out. PNI is one of the emerging interdisciplinary fields being driven by the growing realization that systems cannot be understood in isolation. Simply looking at immunology at the level of the immune cells, neuroscience at the level of neurons, and psychology at the level of behavior and mental states does not capture the complex interactions operating among all these levels. PNI is beginning to shed light on how physical health and the immune system are affected by psychological health. A strong trusting relationship between a doctor and a patient can evoke a positive psychological response in the patient, which a number of researchers assert has a demonstrable benefit to the patient's immune system.

Aware that every patient has within him or her the capacity for self-healing, doctors like Lisa, who are healers in the broadest sense of the word, elicit this life-affirming response in the patient through a kind of receptivity that is too rare among physicians.

A man named Steve came to see me after having been treated by another doctor. I could tell he was wary of me, so I asked him what was on his mind. He had a lot of questions. He asked me a few, and then he looked at me with tears in his eyes and said, "Do you think I'm being a baby?"

Apparently he had voiced these concerns to his previous doctor and been put down. It had really devastated this guy. I felt touched that he felt safe enough to tell me this so early on, and I felt enraged that someone in my field would make any person feel that way.

I told him I didn't think he was a baby at all, that his concerns seemed very reasonable to me and some had simple answers and some didn't, and I would tell him what I could. We clicked after that. He trusted me.

This story demonstrates the power of words, for good or ill. When spoken by a physician, whom we may blindly hold in high esteem, to a patient whose vulnerability is heightened by HIV disease, words are likely to be hung on, reviewed, studied for every nuance. Their effects are lasting. In Steve's case, Lisa was the antidote to the apparently crude remarks of the previous physician. Her clearly genuine desire to relieve Steve's fears and restore his self-respect had to lower his level of stress and strengthen the trust basic to the doctor/patient relationship. It also made it more likely that Steve would follow Lisa's recommendations, medical and otherwise.

Lisa believes in the power of the caring, careful word. Her open conversation coupled with her real concern touches her patients, and sometimes she can see it. She saw it in a man named Robert, whom she describes as "very private" and "who always seemed a little angry." They didn't talk much about personal things, but Lisa knew that he had had to give up his apartment and had moved into Shanti House, a residence for people with AIDS.

This one day he came in for a T-cell count he was really emitting bad vibes and giving me short answers. I was already behind, and part of me thought, "I don't want to deal with this guy. Let's just get through this lab review and get him on," and another part of me thought, "I'm going to be taking care of this man for a while longer, and he's unhappy." So I said, "Robert, you seem really upset and angry. Tell me what's going on."

He just stopped. His face changed, his body posture changed. He didn't say anything. So I said, "These last couple of months have been really rough on you." He nodded and said, "Yeah, it's been hard." That was all. We went on with the appointment.

From then on there was a bond between us—not that we became very close—but just making that acknowledgment of his feelings changed our relationship.

Lisa's words told Robert that she was concerned for his state of mind as much as for the state of his physical health. They also demonstrate the kind of holistic caring she practices, where psychological and spiritual health are given weight along with the physical. Lisa's experience says that there is a fundamental human possibility for healing—psychologically and spiritually, if not always physically—up to and during the process of dying.

There are not enough physicians who count their patients' mental and emotional health as legitimate and vital as their physical health, or who attend to problems other than the physical ones. Those who acknowledge the patients' own capacity for healing, however, tap into those deeper areas of psychospiritual health, for there one may find the peace that heals. This kind of healing is a far cry from the more frequent state of affairs, a rigid and formulaic interaction between doctor and patient in which neither touches the other's humanity, neither affirms the other, and the doctor simply hands down diagnoses, prognoses, and prescriptions from on high, and the patient shuffles off to fulfill them.

Doctors who engage only diseases, not people, are apt to leave their patients feeling frustrated and short-changed regardless of how well they respond to treatment. In fact, care *of* the patient requires caring *for* the patient.

The single most difficult thing for me is the issue of hope and denial. When is it time to direct a person to palliative care? Bernie Siegel [author of *Love, Medicine and Miracles*] says doctors should never tell people how much time they have left. But what if the patient says, "I want to see my mother before I die. How much time do I have?"

I guess the main thing I've learned so far is honesty is the best policy. If I'm not certain, I say it. If I'm uncomfortable talking about something but I think it's important to talk about, I say so. This comes up in discussions about euthanasia all the time.

Though it is an uncomfortably sensitive subject for many care-givers, euthanasia comes up for people with AIDS. Penny Chernow, whose story appears in this book, told me, "Every HIV-positive person I've worked with over the past six years has talked about their suicide kit. When they get too sick and it's just too difficult, they're going to take themselves out."

But very few do. The process of thinking about controlling one's own dying may offer some benefit to the person with AIDS, and understanding that may be helpful to the people who care for them. It's not possible to predict how one will feel later. For some people at the end of their lives, a visit from a friend is worth living for. And for others, nothing is.

Whether to keep up treatments, or switch to a course of care that no longer hopes to cure but only attempts to keep the patient's pain under control is another discussion that is bound to come up, probably more than once, with the patient and/or with the patient's loved ones. Lisa had several such conversations with her patient, Dan.

Dan had a very rough go with his first episode of PCP, so rough that quality of life had become a primary concern to him. When he couldn't speak clearly, communicate clearly, or play the piano, which was the love of his life, he wanted to be allowed to die. We documented all this.

Then he got an abrupt onset illness over a weekend and was admitted to the General. I found out about it on Monday and went to see him. His nurse on the ward said he had been delirious for two days. I held his hand and we chit-chatted, and he'd go off on tangents here and there. So I said, "Dan, I came here to discuss something very important with you, but based on how you are right now, I'm not sure this is the best time."

He looked me straight in the eyes and said, "Oh, you mean the death talk."

I said, yes, that was it, and he said, "You know what I told you in the clinic five months ago, Lisa. I feel the same way now. Please let me go." And I said, "Dan, that's loud and clear." Then he relaxed and went right back into his delirium.

A lot of people didn't believe that he could understand anything I said, or communicate back to me. This experience with Dan and my colleagues' response to it really caught me off guard, and has influenced me a great deal. We sometimes assume that people with mental or psychological impairments can't be reached. But just because their geography isn't navigable most of the time, doesn't mean that it is never navigable.

This is an observation that other caregivers have made in these chapters. Dementia is pierced with lucidity. The caregiver who knows this can make a lasting difference in the life of someone whose world has been altered by this AIDS-related condition. Patients with dementia are often shunned, especially in their dying time; then their physicians become part of an ever smaller circle of caregivers remaining to provide essential care.

Despite his dementia, Lisa trusts that Dan is still the ultimate authority on how he feels and that she will always be at a distance from the center of his experience. So she proceeds as if her partnership with her patient is still intact, but she is honest about her uncertainty, telling Dan outright that she doesn't know if he's in shape to answer her.

The physician who respects her patients, who has a real interest in them, who feels affection for them, who may even leaven
these discussions with humor, supports her patients' dignity and
assures them that they will be cared for always. And supporting
their dignity and offering assurance are healing invocations. While
they may not prevent one's dying, they do help in the deeply personal process of becoming whole psychologically and spiritually.
This is the kind of healing that can continue as long as we live.

－－－

When she's established some rapport with a patient, Lisa feels
comfortable sharing some aspects of her life and herself—where she
and her partner went on vacation, stories about Mason and Dixon,
her two Great Danes, or simply the fact that right now she'd love a
cup of coffee. It's a way she demonstrates her humanness. She wants
her patients to know she is more than "the doctor." It makes her
relationships with them very different.

I've learned it's okay to show feelings, even to cry in front
of patients and their families, because when they know you
care about them, they trust you.
     I've also learned that saying "I don't know" is okay if you
say it right. You can say "I don't know" as in "I don't care," or
"Don't bother me." Or you can say, "I don't know, but I think
it's important. Why don't you do this, and I'll look into that,
and we'll talk about it at your next visit." People really like it
when you say you don't know because it says you're honest
with them.
     Another thing I've learned is how important it is that
things make sense to the patient. We're not taught this in
medical school. If you had PCP, one of the first things I'd
tell you is that you're probably going to have high fevers for
the next four or five days, even if you're doing great, because
that's just the way it is. So when you're burning up and soak-

ing your nightshirt, be frustrated, be angry, but don't be worried.

Sometimes people get bent out of shape over something that doesn't seem like such a big deal, some minor side effect to a drug, say. But maybe their boyfriend had this side effect and died a week later. It's good to try and track the meaning of "overreactions."

✎ ✎ ✎

I'm actually a very compulsive, neurotic doctor, as most internists are. I compile detailed notes about my patients' functional and emotional concerns. I record what the patient is concerned about, like his sexual function, or losing his hair, and what I'm concerned about, like side effects from a drug I'm prescribing or the progress of his KS.

I always begin by asking patients "How are things going?" to let them set the agenda. I have my compulsive checklist, so I can let my stuff wait. I think this sends an important message that this is your illness, not mine.

Communication, open dialogue, as well as subtler messages, as the one above, are for Lisa, part of the practice of medicine. She is also sensitive to the possibility of miscommunication. The patient who is feeling anxious and frightened about what's happening to his body may not be able to say that directly. This patient wants his anxiety addressed, as well as his illness treated. When the doctor responds in the treatment-only mode, the patient may feel frustrated or even angry. So Lisa takes some time and probes a little and tries to draw her patients out—but she wonders at what cost.

I struggle with the issue of efficiency. I usually see three people an hour on follow-up visits. That's much less than most doctors. I tend to see a lot of people for depression, something you'd never uncover unless you talked to them, or spent some quiet time with them where you could pick up their mood.

To do a good job, to have a person feel at ease, you've got to spend time; and at a certain point you may not be reimbursed for that. It's an ethical and personal struggle: how much efficiency can I sacrifice in an operational sense, and still give good care?

✦ ✦ ✦ ✦

I had a patient named Tony who had been sick with a horrible chain of infections. When he was hospitalized, his mother came from New York. She was the prototypical Italian mother, completely devoted and completely torn apart by her inability, and my inability, and probably most horribly God's inability or refusal to make her son better.

She prayed and she went to church and she alternated between being very realistic about how he was doing and saying, "I'm praying for a miracle." Then he got a series of pneumonias and went into multi-organ failure, and she wanted us to put him on dialysis.

But I had promised Tony that I would let him die peacefully when this time came, and I told her that I had to honor my pledge. She was very angry. She said I was preventing God from making a miracle. She said I was killing her son.

I told her that I wanted there to be a miracle for every patient. I said that I had seen many miracles, but these happened when patients and their loved ones learned to be at peace with their suffering and their death. I told her I wished that for her. I hoped by addressing her at a spiritual level that she could connect, but she couldn't.

By this time the nurses on the floor, who had borne the brunt of this mother's misery and concern for over a week, were rolling their eyes, and wishing she would get it together. But I didn't see her as crazy or ridiculous. I saw her trying to deal with a horrible thing, and it happened that the way she dealt with it made it very difficult for us.

I try to look at the bigger picture. I try to think how Tony would like me to be with his mom. I'm taking care of Tony, I'm taking care of his family.

And yet, I was mad at her. I wanted her to let me off the hook, give me her blessing. Not forgive me, necessarily, but let me know she understood. But she never did. Maybe she needed to be mad at me rather than at God.

In one's dying time, the emotional atmosphere may be a force to reckon with as family and loved ones, often with their own unresolved issues, or frustrations, or sadness, or pain, come together for their final visits. It can be an explosive mix, or a roller-coaster ride, or when miracles occur, as Lisa says, it can be a time of peace, solace, and reconciliation.

Here too, the caregiver plays a role. She cares about how her patient is affected, and therefore has a vested interest in how these emotional tides turn. Sometimes she can intercede, sometimes be a conduit for information. Sometimes, as in Tony's case, she can only be her patient's advocate.

Sustained conflict between physicians (or other caregivers) and family members can be a real problem, making it difficult for the person with AIDS to reaffirm the basic meaning and value of his relationships with those around him. Family members, loved ones, and other caregivers can give the dying person a final gift: an atmosphere of support and love that may help lessen the fear and grief of separation. Lisa tries to help create that climate, but it's not always possible.

It's important to remember that anger is a common defense against anxiety and terror. Tony's mother may have believed that accepting his imminent death was somehow pulling against him. Some people think that being realistic about a loved one's dying will cause him or her terrible anguish—they imagine suicide or mental breakdown. These extreme possibilities are often only reflections of their own struggle to face the facts.

Whatever the facts, it is vital that doctors and other caregivers consider the patient *and* the family or network of loved ones as the unit of care, and not just the patient alone; and it is vital that they help provide the family or network full and appropriate support. This is part of the "good care" Lisa fears is often lost to "efficiency."

Tony's nurses rolled their eyes at his difficult mother, but some caregivers go further. Medical professionals are under a lot of pressure themselves, and they're only human. Many would think, "I'm working my butt off for your son and you give me this crap—I don't have to take it. I'm out of here." And without ever saying those words out loud, they would essentially withdraw emotionally, maybe physically too. No one would say anything. It would never be acknowledged or addressed. But the nurses would know and other people watching would know that the doctor is no longer fully involved.

Another all too common response is to disqualify the distraught person's reality by labeling it irrational or hysterical or otherwise abnormal. This is frequently less an objective assessment than a reflection of the caregiver's own inability to cope with intense emotional or behavioral responses. In fact, as many of us know, unusual behavior and intense emotion may make absolute sense in the unusual and intense times that AIDS enscribes.

◢◢◢◢

While patients frequently affirm the major role nurses play in their ability to cope and improve, and recognize the powerful healing force of their nurses' knowledge and compassionate care, physicians rarely do. An exception is author/physician Lewis Thomas, who wrote of nurses in *The Youngest Science*, "If they ask for the moon, I am on their side." Lisa is another exception.

I've learned from the nurses I work with that I can be emotionally open. Every two weeks I have a two-hour meeting with the nurses who take care of my homecare patients. It's ostensibly a case management meeting to go over the patients they see. Every once in a while I give a talk about antibiotics, or CMV, or something technical. But most important to us is telling stories, about the hard things, or fun things, and every once in a while it totally degenerates into teenage humor. It's a place where we can let it all hang out.

When those two weeks are up, I'm ready. It's like we're all on this life raft together. We counsel and support each other. So many of these nurses have so much more experience than I have. I tell them something and they say, "That was a hard choice. I think you did the best anyone could do." It means a tremendous amount to me.

They've taught me that it's okay to be a mush ball. That you can be completely mad at a patient and still take good care of him. We've also talked a lot about spiritual stuff around our work, which, my God, is unheard of! About finding meaning in our work, times when you have a clinical situation that's just a mess with everybody butting heads, and all of a sudden a moment of peace happens. Or being with a patient when she dies, or talking to a patient about dying. These epiphanies. It's nice to be able to talk about these things.

Lisa's respect for the nurses she works with as colleagues and teachers is unusual, and it speaks to her belief in a collaborative model of caregiving. More common is the rigidly hierarchical model that calls the physician the boss and the nurse a subordinate. When caregiving is based on a foundation of dominance at this level, I believe it is the patient, at the bottom of the ladder, who is the ultimate loser.

✔ ✔ ✔

I had a patient named Richard who was semiconscious. I'd go in to see him some days and not have any sense of us connecting, and yet I persisted in putting down the bed rails and talking with him. I'm sure the nurses thought I was crazy talking to this guy and telling him what we were doing, but it seemed like the right thing to do.

I think of it this way: if this were my grandmother lying here, I would want her doctor to put down the bed rail and talk to her. I call this the Grandmother Principle. I find it a really nice centering rule. Those times I wonder why I have to explain this procedure to the family again, or fill out this paperwork, I think of my grandmother and how I'd want her doctor to treat her family respectfully and see to her paperwork.

The more I do this medical work, the more I think of her. She died when I was sixteen, so it's been a while. Both my mother's and father's parents immigrated from Italy not speaking a word of English, yet they managed to start businesses and make it through really rough times. I hope I inherited a little of their pioneer spirit.

It's a good image for Lisa, a pioneer caregiver for collaborative healing, where trusting and working closely with one's patients allows them to invoke the physician's strength and their own as allies in their struggle to survive with AIDS.

9
I Listen to
Each Person's Truth

My parents raised us in California to escape the racism and poverty of the South, but they brought their fears and hurts with them along with their hopes, and we all lived with them. I learned how to armor myself and protect myself from the worst and not let the rest matter. It was wounding with love, but it was wounding.

Growing up in a Creole family (mixed black, white, and Indian ancestry) in a largely Caucasian town, Eric Poche learned the value of discretion and of silence; but he was too intelligent and too creative to deny communication. He learned to "develop a language of feelings, where you realize that you can communicate and sense things other than with words." That language has served him well in his work with people with AIDS.

In high school, Eric's guidance counselor asked him what he wanted to do with his future, and Eric replied, "I'd really like to help people—to make a difference." The counselor responded with a sarcastic, "Well, isn't *that* nice." Eric's dream dissolved. He went on to college, but didn't pursue a helping profession. He earned a bachelor of arts degree, moved to San Francisco, and took a position with a British-owned corporation. Almost twenty years later he reclaimed his heart's desire when he volunteered to provide practical support for people with AIDS through Shanti Project.

Shanti and other AIDS agencies have found it useful to allow volunteers to choose between providing clients with practical or emotional support. Those who offer emotional support act as peer counselors, nonjudgmental, active listeners to whom the client may talk about the fears, hopes, and problems that are part of living with HIV disease. Those who volunteer practical support go grocery shopping, clean, cook, do the laundry, write letters for the client, and try in these and other utilitarian ways to provide for his or her physical comfort.

With my first client, Robbie, who was pretty much bedbound, I followed all the rules. Six hours a week, that's it, you go home. I'd bring him breakfast, we'd sit and eat together, and then I'd clean, launder, or shop for him. But for me it was more than buying the groceries and bringing them home and putting them on the table. I'd buy a chicken. I'd skin it and season it and wrap the extra pieces and freeze them. I wanted to do more than just get what Robbie needed. I wanted to make things as easy and comfortable for him as possible.

His appetite was very poor. When his Open Hand meals began stacking up in the refrigerator, I decided he needed some chicken soup. He had difficulty with fats, so I skimmed the fat off the top, and I seasoned it just right. There I was in the kitchen just humming away. When I brought him that bowl of soup he said, "This is good. You know, I think you just saved my life."

Eric's acts of service are performed like meditations. That he takes great pleasure in preparing food with his client's specific needs as the crucial ingredient is clear when we picture him humming away in Robbie's kitchen. That pleasure communicates to his clients. The chores are concrete gestures of Eric's devotion, and as such, no matter how apparently modest the tasks—folding towels, watering plants, seasoning soup—they carry with them the elements of devotion: allegiance, dependability, trustworthiness, affection.

In relating to his clients, Eric projects a calm, steadying influence. He is a thoughtful, careful man who rarely overreacts to the dramas that are part of life in the world of AIDS caregiving. He regards the best caregiving as neither complex nor dramatic. It is a simple matter, in his belief, of one's unadorned presence, and one's honest intention to do the best possible job for the client.

I called Robbie to see how he was doing, and he told me his feet had been irradiated again and they were all scabbed over and it was very difficult for him to walk. This was weeks after the treatment. Very hesitantly, he said, "I could use some slippers." So I went and bought slippers two sizes too big so he could get his feet into them. I didn't make an issue of any of it.

✦ ✦ ✦ ✦

As practical caregivers, we bring *ourselves* as well as our scouring pads and laundry soap and shopping carts into the lives of our clients. No matter what service the caregiver is performing, he or she is *there* for the client, is the difference between no one and someone. The two establish a relationship in which there is plenty of emotional content—the bond between a client and his or her practical support volunteer is often as strong as between the client and the caregiver who volunteers emotional support. To my knowledge no practical caregiver has ever said, "I'm sorry, I only make soup and change diapers, I don't discuss hopes and fears." Hopes and fears, uncertainty and urgency, and heart to hearts are part of the territory when you live with AIDS or care for people with

AIDS. There is frequently no way to separate the physical from the emotional aspects of a life-threatening illness, and no way not to get involved with aspects of both when you care for people with AIDS, regardless of how you care for them.

As with other relationships, it takes a while to develop the caregiving partnership. Especially in the case of practical caregiving, the client may have deep feelings of conflict: gratitude for your good samaritan service, shame or regret at not being able to do for himself:

> In the beginning Robbie would say, "Thank you for coming," and then he would turn away. But eventually he realized that I was there because I cared. I cared about his comfort. I left evidence of that.
>
> It's important not to have expectations that a person is going to be appreciative or respond to you the way you expect. I was alert to the gradual shifting, where he began to ask me questions about myself, where he began to understand and accept that I would do this or that and that I didn't see these things as problems and that *we* could handle it.
>
> One time he said to me, "I've just had a movement," meaning diarrhea. I took what I hoped was a discreet deep breath, and said quietly, "Well, let's clean it up." What followed was a slow process of changing, cleaning, washing, powdering, and replacing the linen with Robbie directing every step, very much involved and expressive.
>
> Previously I'd only shaken his hand or touched him on the shoulder. It was important for me not to infantilize him in any way so he would feel enabled, not simply done for.

✐ ✐ ✐

When AIDS causes someone to require a practical caregiver, the recipient may be spending a great deal of time alone and may be feeling desperately cut off, unheard, invisible. Because there's no one to talk to, the isolated individual often turns inward, looking for comfort if not company in a smaller and smaller world of experience. Thus the inwardly focused individual further isolates himself from the possibility of discovering love or companionship from someone outside. He becomes almost a prisoner of his own existence. It is in such situations that caregivers like Eric often manifest their greatest gifts.

Billie was in his mid-twenties, an IV drug user, and a transsexual whose milieu was Polk Street [an area in San Francisco known for its young hustlers and drug culture]. He was having injections so he was growing breasts. He was incredibly proud of them. He loved to feel them wobbling. He used to run around the house wearing pearls and that's all, with his hair teased to death shouting, "I'm becoming WOMAN!" Billie was someone I would probably never have known outside of AIDS work.

I'm sure he thought, "This person has an education, this person is older, this person has a good job and all these interests—how can we relate?"

Even though we came from such different worlds, there was an area where we communicated, and that was in laughter. Billie had a wonderful laugh where you could hear the joy behind it. It lifted you up to hear it, whether you knew what was so funny or not. It became very important to allow that laughter a place to come out because he was struggling with so much. I gave him that place.

But I didn't want to be around him if he was using [drugs]. It was part of our agreement that I always call before I came over to make sure he wasn't loaded. Then one day he told me he wanted to stop using. He wanted to do it for his family. He didn't want to die still using. And I said, "Have you thought about getting some help or support for that?" And he became livid. He said, "You're here to help me clean the house. You're not here to give me advice." So I went back into the kitchen.

Billie had a problem with cockroaches. I decided that now was the time to do what I had avoided doing for weeks, and that was to clean behind the refrigerator. When I moved the refrigerator a carpet of cockroaches scattered everywhere. I went at it with cleaner, ammonia, the whole business, just scrubbing away like a mad thing.

He came into the kitchen and told me I didn't have to be doing that, and I said, "I'm doing it because I think it might be a little healthier for you." And he said, "I'm going to bed."

Billie would do that sometimes, go to bed and pull the covers over his head. He was very angry with me for suggesting he couldn't get off drugs alone. But I just finished my business, and called goodbye to him, and left. It's like Micaela says, "You show up, you pay attention, and you care."

Eric's very presence suggested that there was much that Billie couldn't do alone. But verbalizing it crossed a line for Billie. No matter how well-intentioned Eric's remark, it did not have the desired effect, to encourage and support Billie in his wish to quit using drugs.

Society has taught drug users like Billie to judge themselves very harshly. The constant message of how they *should* be makes it tough to accept themselves as they are—as people, not just users. It's not uncommon then, to turn one's anger and frustration and disappointment inward, and engage in constant, chronic self-criticism that seems escapable only through more drug use.

Billie may have been an old pro at self-criticism, but apparently he was not in shape to deal with Eric's suggestion that he might not be capable of self-control. Even if it was true. Especially if it was true. In Billie's mind, Eric's words conveyed judgment and denigration. And this from one of the few people Billie was beginning to think he could count on, who didn't seem to make any judgments.

So Billie lashed out. Caregivers will learn that anger is frequently a defense against fear and loss of control. Active listening—with one's head and heart to the words the client uses, to the actions that accompany the words—makes it easier to understand this. The emotional realities of living with AIDS are different from those in the world without AIDS. For people with AIDS, anger can sometimes be a psychologically adaptive and emotionally healthy response to severe stress. It can also feel manipulative and hurtful to the recipient.

In the face of Billie's angry response, Eric, who is surely one of the most gracious individuals under fire, retreated immediately, and retrenched by tackling a practical, if odious job. Going back to the basic contract of practical support helped reestablish some equilibrium in the situation. Billie may have drawn the covers over his head, but at some level he understood the meaning of Eric's gesture.

Billie called me the next week and asked to come visit me at my apartment, which he had never done before. I had tea and cookies for us and we sat and talked, and then he walked around my apartment and said, "This is a really nice place. I'll never have a place like this."

I reminded him that he had a place, and that we could take care of it, and that seemed to inspire him, and he began to talk about things he'd like to do, and one of them was to cook a pot roast that we would share. This was a man who had lived his life on the streets as a hustler, who had thrown away the past he'd grown up with to live this way, and he was dreaming about pot roast. We knew it would never happen, but we also knew that this was something he really wanted to believe, so for that moment we believed it together.

In a sense, it was an elaborate test Billie had designed for Eric, but so far Eric was passing with flying colors. First he had allowed Billie to vent his anger and he did not quit, and his attitude toward Billie didn't seem to have been damaged or changed in any way. Then he had let Billie into his own home. And then he had stepped into Billie's fantasy world with him, a world where pot roast symbolized the warmth of family, hearth, and home.

I had some Mardi Gras beads that Billie fell in love with:
three sets—one silver, one dark gray, one mauve. Before
he left, I told him to take the strand he liked best. I thought
he would take the silver, but he chose the dark gray. He
hugged me very tightly that day, and said, "I never want us
to be angry with each other. I wouldn't hurt you for anything."

The next week I called him as usual, but all I got was a
busy signal. Sometimes he took his phone off the hook when
he wanted to nap. I figured he was home, so I went over.
He didn't answer the doorbell, but the lights were on inside,
so I went in, and there was Billie, in his pearls and not much
else, dead. There was shit all over the place. He'd OD'd,
and panicked probably, and just shit everywhere. He had
two cats. I found them in the closet, terrified.

I took a deep breath and replaced the phone in its cradle.
It was covered with excrement. Maybe he was trying to phone
for help. I locked the apartment and went across the street
and called 911. I was just barely holding it together.

The ambulance responded very quickly. The coroner was
pulling on his latex gloves and they were stretching tape to
cordon off the apartment by the time I got back, and it all
turned very official. "Who are you? What's your relationship
here? Did you call this in?" Suddenly my job was over because
Billie wasn't there. To this day I wish that I had sat with him
a little longer before going to make that call.

━ ━ ━

Billie had a truth. And that's what I value. Sometimes
it's not an easy truth to be with, sometimes it's very illusive,
sometimes it's piled over with stuff and you can't see it, but
it's there.

When people talk to you they're telling you their truth.
Sometimes it's blatant and unvarnished, but rarely, I think,
because people don't usually trust that much—especially
strangers. But people will tell you a story, and in it is a grain

of truth and a reason why it has to be told. I try to remember to listen for that.

Eric's assumption that people are always trying to communicate their truth to us is one that can be very useful to caregivers. We should be aware that this kind of communication may occur in ways other than speech, and that even a verbal expression of truth may be symbolic, as in Billie's fantasy about pot roast. Sometimes a person communicates with silence. Billie's crawling under the covers seems to say, "Intimacy frightens me. I'm growing more dependent on you and I need to get away." Sometimes a person communicates with rage. But Billie's angry outburst—"You're here to help me clean . . . not give advice"— sends the same message about intimacy as his silence did.

Caregivers who are not professional psychotherapists or counselors can't be expected to interpret nuances of communication with great sophistication or accuracy, but it is helpful to consider that whatever our clients say or don't say, they will try to tell us something essential about themselves.

Some mental health professionals emphasize the opposite: that people like Billie are in fact trying to hide the truth about themselves, or deny it. Some psychotherapists may spend precious months engaged in a battle of wits with a client, trying to get to the bottom of things, to discover cause and motivation—when useful truths lie closer to the surface, and come up in more than one way, and come up repeatedly—if we only knew how to read them. Also, it's my experience that using lengthy intellectualized psychotherapeutic approaches with a client for the purpose of revealing hidden truths may actually obscure those truths and distance the caregiver emotionally from the client.

✒ ✒ ✒

Eric has worked full time as a volunteer coordinator for Shanti Project for several years. He is also an artist and craftsman, designing and executing detailed woodblock prints. One of my favorites is entitled, "Epidemic Cares," in which shapes vaguely like human beings seem trapped under layers of debris, above which float other humanoid shapes. To me, the print speaks of liberation, and of Eric's ability to approach complex issues with simple but potent statements that need not be made with words.

As the sole survivor of his second circle of gay friends, ongoing mourning and protracted pain have had a significant impact on Eric. Grieving lost loved ones has led him to question the role of intimacy in the era of AIDS. In what ways is a life commitment to caregiving a healthy form of intimacy? Or is such a commitment really a form of psychological defense that people living in the throes of a pandemic use to protect themselves against further emotional upheaval in their personal lives? We'll need a better understanding of the impact of the AIDS pandemic on human relationships before we can answer these questions. We do know that unusual styles of coping, and unique adaptations, occur in life in extremity, and that those choices we make in a plague may not resemble choices we would make in healthy times.

> What I'm working on being clear about for myself is that my caregiving is not a substitution for something else. I don't want it to preclude other options, other ways of thinking or feeling. I feel as if I need to look at what intimacy means to me, and how I can have that in conjunction with caregiving, or is it always going to be second to my involvement in caregiving? I don't know the answers to these questions.

Eric has mastered one of the most essential aspects of intimacy: small, uncomplicated gestures that require only a modicum of effort, but make a big statement because of how genuine they are. His actions say plainly, "I won't let you down." He also knows the value of the loving touch, another aspect of intimacy that requires little effort. Eric is famous for his all-encompassing embrace, a way he communicates a truth about himself to his friends and his clients—which is how much he loves us, and how much he himself needs love.

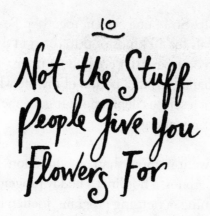

10
Not the Stuff People Give you Flowers For

It's kind of scary how I became an AIDS "expert." I was working with St. Louis Effort for AIDS in 1985, and I was the only person who was willing to use my whole name when the media came looking for someone to interview.

Joellen Sheerin, R.N., had been working as a primary care nurse in a large St. Louis hospital in 1983 when she encountered her first patient with AIDS. At that time no one knew how AIDS was transmitted. Joellen had to don "Martian garb" to care for him.

She volunteered to help organize the first agency response to AIDS in St. Louis. "I thought I'd do my little bit for AIDS and scoot off the stage," Joellen told me. Instead, she became a media personality and public speaker on behalf of St. Louis Effort for AIDS. She also developed their volunteer training model, based on literature Shanti Project in San Francisco sent her. Because she was a nurse, she became Effort for AIDS's lead case manager.

Nobody knew who the clients were, nobody knew who had AIDS in the city, what services were available, who was

willing to help. So I put a system together. People would
call for referrals for all kinds of things, and I'd direct them
to the person or group that could help them.

This all happened in a period of my life when I was just
coming out of a serious depression. It gave me a direction,
a place to put my energy.

That energy went in more than one direction. Effort for AIDS
included support groups, a hot line, a buddy program, financial aid,
and in the beginning, a housing program. Joellen became a member of the board of directors, and then its treasurer. A whole new
Joellen began to emerge:

I did a lot of TV talk shows, a lot of community education.
I really loved it. I'd never done anything like it in my life.
I'd just been a floor nurse in intensive care. Public speaking—I found I was really good at it, and good at organizing
things.

She spent the next three and a half years volunteering with St.
Louis Effort for AIDS. After a vacation to San Francisco in 1989,
she decided to make AIDS caregiving her full-time work. She
applied and was accepted at San Francisco General Hospital, and
moved to California in 1990.

╸╸╸╸

The serious depression that Joellen was pulling out of when she
began her AIDS caregiving was a legacy of what she described as
"an alcoholic and sexually abusive father." She thought that getting
away from home, moving into her own apartment after nursing
school, would end her problems, but it didn't.

I hurt so bad all the time, I couldn't stand it. One night I
couldn't think of any reason why I should go on living.

Then my two kittens walked into the room, and I realized there'd be no one to take care of them if I killed myself. My two cats occupy a cherished position in my home today.

A seminar on incest and child abuse became the catalyst for Joellen's recovery. Part of what influenced her to move to San Francisco was the possibility of finding a therapist to help her work on these issues, which she has been successful in doing. She attributes some of her talent as a caregiver to her painful past. "I think I'm particularly sensitive to people with AIDS because I spent so much time knowing that no one could help me, no one could make it better or make it go away."

＊＊＊＊

I took care of Tom several times over the course of his illness. He had AIDS dementia, and was often in some kind of psychotic state, but he really liked me, and I really liked him, too. On his last admission, he no longer spoke in sentences, but in strings of words.

He had herpes on his butt and he had had an attack of diarrhea. I was cleaning him up, but because of the sores it was painful for him, and out of the string of words came "Nazi woman from hell . . ." I felt so awful. I said, "Oh my God, Tom, I'm really sorry it hurts; I'm just trying to help you."

Dementia patients are a lot of times the hardest to take care of. You're not sure what they're perceiving. I didn't want Tom to think I would hurt him. After we finished cleaning up, I said, "Tom, do you know who I am?" And he said, "Yeah. Pink woman, soft hugs."

Joellen identifies strongly with her role as a nurturing caregiver. It's painful to her to be thought of as someone who pokes, prods, and causes another to suffer. She helps us understand the distinction between "cure," the more objective aspects of diagnosing and treating a disease, and "care," which has more to do with the subjective meanings for the patient of the disease and its treatment. Curing activities require that Joellen do things *to* her patient. It is when she cares *for* that she can do things *with* the patient, and this aspect of nursing provides her the greatest gratification. Joellen demonstrates that she cares by reaching out—literally:

> I was really glad that the way I show I care had stuck with Tom. I know some people aren't comfortable with hugs, but a lot of times they want to be hugged. Especially when there's nothing I can say to them, a hug will let them know I care about them.

Joellen's challenge, and that of other caregivers, is to be tough on problems and tender on people. Severely limiting one's emotional accessibility, restricting interaction with patients to efficiency-geared behaviors designed to "cure," may instead cause needless suffering. How often have we seen health professionals argue with a patient for precious minutes about the necessity of a procedure, when investing the same amount of time listening to the patient's concerns and answering them was the more productive road? Many patient-caregiver arguments in these cases are clashes over who's in charge of what happens to the patient. Such a battle compromises both caregiver task-efficiency and patient well-being.

> I had a patient who was pretty good during the day, but at night she'd pull out her IVs and get out of bed and try to walk around. I had to put her in a restraining jacket at night and tie her into bed. In the morning the day nurse took her out of the jacket. The next night she said, "I know you hate me," when I began to tie her down.
> I told her that I didn't hate her. I just didn't know what to do with her, and I sat down next to the bed and talked

to her for a few minutes. I said, "Look at your arm. You see how it's bleeding? That's because you were just up and in the bathroom and you forgot you have all these IVs. You don't have a lot of places to put IVs, and I have to keep redoing them, and then you pull everything out. I don't want you to hurt yourself." We both cried. I think she really understood.

When I've taken the time to sit and talk to somebody and really explain where I'm coming from and why I'm doing these awful things to them, we both feel better. Because a lot of times what I do to people isn't fun stuff. It's not the stuff people give you flowers for.

~~~~

The kind of caregiving that nurses do often takes place in a hierarchically based organization where nurses, and everybody else, are intensely aware of who's got power over whom. In these organizations, the sad truth is that the individual at the bottom of the hierarchy, the one with the least power of all, is the patient. This model of care views patients as if they were machines with broken parts or other system damage, and health care professionals as if they were mechanics. While the mechanics repair their machines' malfunctions, they don't expect the machines to give them a bad time, to talk back, or to make demands.

Professional caregivers are hardly to blame. They have been trained in this system, taught to deal with diseases, not with people. Part of what's wrong with the current model is the mistaken idea that there is one right course of treatment for a person's particular disease, instead of acknowledgment that no two people respond to the same treatment, intervention, or situation in the same way.

In many organizations nurses are severely overburdened, and not just by the number of tasks they must perform for one patient after another. Many believe that they should be able to take care of all their patients' needs if they only work harder or assume greater responsibility. In fact, they are striving to become better nurses by becoming more efficient mechanics. They lay down the ground rules for their patients: "You cooperate with me, and I'll smile at you and get through this list of things I have to do in this certain amount of time. But if you're going to give me a hard time, there'll be repercussions."

Anyone who works with educated gay men with AIDS or streetwise IV drug users will soon discover that the downside of this approach is resentment, alienation, even despair on the part of the client or patient.

The machine model is severely limited. And for years, health professionals have been pointing a finger at one another and at their administrations, to lay the blame for its failure—to no avail. It is something intrinsic to the model that's at fault. Its premises of dominance and hierarchy have subverted our best efforts at a human-centered model for health care, where the patient whose overall welfare is the primary concern of this web of caregiving relationships occupies the central position, and caregivers radiate from that center. But in the absence of such a model or support for one, hyperstressed, overburdened caregivers fall back on their old ways of coping with assigned tasks and the emotions that bubble up when you're dealing with patient needs and professional responsibilities. And these are the ways of power and hierarchy that require patient obedience and compliance—or else. In the case of a vulnerable patient with AIDS, the implicit "or else" is the ultimate threat of force or abandonment.

For nurses and other professionals who are committed to a different style of care based on a human-centered model that addresses the psychosocial, emotional, and spiritual needs of people with AIDS, I offer these guidelines:

1. With the patient, define major areas of distress.

2. Respond to the patient's requests for information as completely and accurately as you can.

3. Be honest with the patient's loved ones about the patient's health status as it changes.

4. Describe staff expectations regarding treatment and patient-staff relationships to the patient, and elicit the patient's expectations as well.

5. It's hazardous to make unilateral judgments about another person's emotional reality. Always compare your perceptions of what's going on with what the patient, the patient's loved ones, and your colleagues think is going on.

6. Remember that psychosocial evaluation, like medical and nursing appraisal, is a continuous process that requires far more time and skill than most case conferences and staff meetings demonstrate.

- - - -

The other day, I had to say goodbye to a patient, Richard, who was on his way to the hospice. It's so hard, because you want to send them off happy, but you can't. You can't even pretend you're going to see them again. There are no words to make it better. So I just sat with Richard, and said, "I'm really sorry you're so sick," and he said, "I thought I had more time."

Those are the times it's awful when you really care about somebody.

Joellen's story demonstrates her willingness to accept her own strong emotional responses as an integral part of her work. It is a great benefit for AIDS caregivers to know that such feelings and reactions as sadness, or depression, or anger, are as normal as feelings of satisfaction in relation to their work.

When caregivers believe certain emotions are unacceptable or a sign of weakness, and when the work setting does not provide avenues of support for emotional expression (such as support groups and/or readily available professional consultations), then their evolution as caregivers and as human beings is undermined.

Emotions are information about ourselves. When we are discouraged from exploring this vital side of our human nature, and are encouraged to suppress our emotions, we are simultaneously encouraged to deny or hide our needs rather than to express them. When we habitually ignore our own psychosocial and emotional needs, we invite severe stress, and in response to such stress we sometimes try to protect ourselves against genuine person-to-person encounters with our clients or patients. Many caregivers do this by withdrawing from their patients, although they may be quite unaware of it. Following are examples of that kind of withdrawal:

1. Referring to the patient as a disease or unit of service: "The KS lesions in the waiting room." "The PCP in room 43." This is the caregiver's unconscious effort to sidestep his or her own difficulty in managing feelings by objectifying the patient and the situation.

2. Cynicism about psychosocial and emotional needs in general. Taking the position that a stiff upper lip is preferable to "sharing." Perfunctory questions may be evidence of this kind of cynicism. For instance, health care professionals know that the question, "How are you doing?" is likely to elicit the one word answer, "Fine," whether the patient is fine or not. (I've only heard one patient respond differently. To his nurse's "How're you doing?" he replied, "I'll be damned if I'll tell my feelings to someone who makes two-minute U-turns at the foot of my bed.")

3. Entering the room without knocking, scheduling procedures unilaterally, limiting visitors intransigently are all actions that say the patient's privacy, needs, and desires are less important than hospital routine.

4. Focusing on technical tasks involving machinery or equipment to the exclusion of the patient. More than one patient

has complained to me that their nurses make more eye contact with the IVs than with the patient.

◢ ◢ ◢

Such avoidance mechanisms actually reduce the caregiver to a dispenser of technical information and procedure. In an attempt to protect ourselves from the feelings that arise in a genuine encounter with our client or patient, we withhold parts of ourselves that can be vitally important in the healing relationship. Maybe we fear the real or imagined enormity of the patient's feelings. Maybe we are afraid that we cannot live up to his or her expectations, or that we lack the skill or the time to address these feelings. Maybe the fear is that our own strong feelings will overwhelm us.

Whatever the basis of caregiver fears, when we deny the patient access to a full human-to-human relationship, we deny something genuinely therapeutic as well. A relationship in which life and death issues are common currency between caregiver and patient is one in which the caregiver may heal and grow along with those for whom he or she cares.

◢ ◢ ◢

Scott was one of my best friends whom I met shortly after I moved to San Francisco. We bonded from the first time we laid eyes on each other. He had been a chef in Italy for some years, and I loved to cook—we had a lot in common. I knew he was HIV positive and had KS, but he hadn't been hospitalized yet.

We talked through a lot of stuff over coffee at Cafe Flore— different kinds of treatments, what he would do and not do. He expected to come to Ward 5A when he got sick, and I promised he wouldn't have to eat the food there and that I would take care of him. It was quite a shock for both of us when I realized that I couldn't.

I wanted to be his friend when he got sick, and not his nurse. I didn't want to get into fights with him about taking his medicine or changing IVs—Scott was deathly afraid of needles. I wanted to be the one he could tell about how awful those nurses were to him, not the one doing those awful things. It was real important to me.

He was mad at first, but we worked it out, and I'm glad we did because a week after that conversation he was in the hospital with CMV retinitis. He had been seeing these little flickers of light for a while, but when I had asked him if he'd had his eyes checked for CMV, he told me no. Someone in his healing group had told him that those flickers were "house fairies." I said, Fine. I think he really appreciated that I let him be—to believe in fairies, to drink his hideous bark tea. I could do that because I wasn't his nurse.

When Scott got admitted, we had his food brought in. He ordered through Waiters on Wheels. I spent time with him as a friend, and since I was working nights, I always said goodnight to him; and I'd say goodbye in the morning if he was awake. I never did take care of him.

And then he died. It was so sudden. I hadn't had time to shift gears, to prepare. But so many times I've sat at memorial services where people say such wonderful things about someone who's died, and I've wondered, "Did the person you're talking about know how you felt?" So often they don't. So I had written Scott this long list of things that I'll always remember about him, and I gave it to him before he went blind from CMV: making tea in a china pot, using fresh basil leaves on sliced tomatoes for a salad, going to the nursery in Half Moon Bay and then having fish and chips at Princeton Seafood Company. Putting lavender in the sheets. The day we spent watching the birds on the waves. Him saying that he'd always keep an eye on me.

━ ━ ━ ━

Joellen demonstrates her understanding that the quality of care she offers any of her patients, including Scott, is a function of her own psychological state as much as her technical expertise. Being close friends with a person for whom you are also professionally responsible doesn't occur all that often, and straddling both roles can be quite a balancing act—between the incessant repetitious routine of hospital nursing, and making time for listening, speaking, and acting from the heart. "It's one thing if someone comes in and I don't know him, and I have to lay down the rules," she told me. "It's another thing if it's my friend."

I think Joellen made the right choice in holding her friendship with Scott sacrosanct and not jeopardizing it by changing their loving relationship to that of a patient and his nurse.

Her story also demonstrates the lack of any forum in the hospital setting for caregivers to deal with the losses that are so much a part of their work. It's a shame when we have to rely exclusively on our own resources in coping with the death of someone we've grown close to. I have been an active advocate for many years of common sense psychosocial support for caregivers who work with seriously ill people. It's not *just* important for the caregiver. Our ability to talk with our clients and patients about living with AIDS and dying from it grows in direct proportion to our ability to share our own anxieties with one another. Don't be shy about seeking a group to share your feelings with. The more we learn to talk honestly together, the more we can bear each other's pain, and our own.

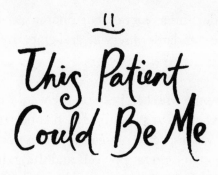

11

This Patient Could Be Me

I remember when I first started as a Shanti counselor working on the AIDS ward at San Francisco General Hospital, and I sat in Report day after day listening to the rundown on patients: "Patient X in Room One has herpes simplex virus, CMV retinitus, no support, homeless. Patient Y in Room Two has KS lesions and neuropathy. Patient Z in Three is a heroin addict with pneumocystis carinii pneumonia and dementia," and on and on. Forty patients in a row. I was exhausted by the end of the report, and I hadn't left the charting room yet. It was like watching a massive tidal wave called AIDS moving in. And there was not very much at all I could do about it but put one foot in front of the other. And that's all I've ever felt like I could do—just keep putting one foot in front of the other.

Bharat Lindemood brings a sensitivity to his AIDS caregiving that comes from his own status as a man with AIDS and years spent cultivating his psyche and his soul through psychological self-inquiry and spiritual practice. For those with whom he works, he is a role model and a teacher, but Bharat says that he doesn't always meet the standards of service and empathy that he has set for himself.

> There was a man who had been on the ward a number of times, and when he was healthier he had been pretty anti-social—he was suspected of stealing things from the unit, like people's coats and tape players and things like that. I avoided him. Eventually he got sicker and developed dementia, and one day he was on my scheduled rounds.
>
> I went into his room thinking, I hope this will be brief. Actually, he was very pleasant. He was watching TV. And as I have done sometimes when I really want to get out of a room, I asked him, "Is there anything I can do for you?" Most of the time people will say no, and you can escape. But he said, "I could really use a video." And I said, "What kind would you like?" And he said, "I'll go with you."
>
> He could barely walk, and the video library was a very long hallway away. And I was impatient to get there and get this man his video so that I could go on to the next patient on my rounds, and feel as if I'd seen a large number of patients that day, and therefore been very helpful.
>
> We finally picked out a couple of videos. I walked him back, got it set up, and I thought, Thank God that's over. And I went on and did my other things.
>
> Two weeks later, his mother came from Central America to visit him, and once again he was on my rounds. When I walked into his room, he said to his mother, "Mom, this is the guy I was telling you about that helped me get the video."

The littlest things mean a lot. This is one of the hardest lessons for caregivers to learn. Your response to the smallest request, to what seems like the most insignificant gesture, is an act that may have untold repercussions for your client. Bharat says, "You can't underestimate the value of opening a window, changing the channel for someone, or just sitting with someone, not even talking."

✐ ✐ ✐

Bharat was drawn to work with terminally ill people in the early 1980s. At around the same time, his mother, who had suffered a number of "nervous breakdowns," committed suicide. Eight years later he and his father became estranged and stopped seeing one another.

After a stint in the Peace Corps in Africa in 1983, he pursued a master's degree in psychology, and went to work in intensive care psychiatric hospitals. He remembers one locked ward on which 90 percent of the patients had histories of violence. He told me he had been wary of the staff and how they would treat their patients more than he worried about the patients themselves, but "I saw that the staff were incredibly compassionate, and that they really respected the patients. They showed me how to make contact with people. Their concern really moved me."

Bharat's commitment to people in psychological and physical distress shifted to people with AIDS when, in 1985, in his mid-twenties, he received his own HIV+ diagnosis. I asked him, "How did your diagnosis of HIV move you to become an AIDS caregiver?"

I'm very much counterphobic—that is, I'm a person who seeks out what he's afraid of in order to stare it in the face.

Can you talk about what you're afraid of?

One of my worst fears was that I would lose my mind, and that as a result of that, people would treat me like I didn't exist anymore. I saw something like this happen with a man who had PML. He started out as this gregarious former bartender whose friends all came to visit with a strong smell of alcohol on their breaths. It wasn't my scene at all. They would come in and I would leave.

As things progressed, he lost control of his extremities, and then he had this muscular deadening in his throat—even his respiration became suppressed. He could no longer talk and he often sat kind of looking into space. But I noticed his eyes tracked people when they came into his room, and he was aware of his environment. But everyone treated him like he was gone already.

I felt helpless with him. What do you do with a person who can't talk to you in the conventional way? I mean, you feel awfully stupid saying, "I care," to someone like that. All those interventions I'd learned didn't seem relevant.

One day, I don't know why, I walked into his room and sat down next to his bed and said, "You know, just because you don't have your old personality doesn't mean we can't hang out together."

His eyes opened and he looked at me with tears in them. My own eyes filled with tears. I didn't have to say anything else. We just hung out there for a while.

Bharat went on to say that "our personalities aren't the only link in this game. . . . Just because you lose your mind doesn't mean you're not there anymore." He has had enough contact with people who have lost their whole personalities through dementia to know that they still may be reached with a caring touch and a loving or supportive presence. Many other caregivers know the same, which is reassuring to Bharat, and has helped him cope with his worst fears.

✦ ✦ ✦

Bharat began caring for people with AIDS in 1985 in Seattle. He moved to San Francisco and came to work for Shanti in 1989 as a counselor on the AIDS ward at San Francisco General. One of the first times he was assigned to work with a man with dementia

THIS PATIENT COULD BE ME   143

and a psychiatric history that included violent and antisocial behavior, part of him wanted to avoid the patient. But another part said, "I have experience working with these kinds of people. Why don't I just go sit in the room and see what happens?"

By walking into a room with his eyes and ears and heart open, even though he's not sure what to expect, Bharat is able to make a connection with the person behind the "dementia" label. This ability, in Bharat's case, seems to come from his skill as a clinician and his compassion for people. He has thought about the word *compassion*. He knows it means to "suffer with," to make an imaginative connection with the world of another's pain, to bridge the distance between the other person's hurt and his own emotional wounds.

> I went in there and the patient was very agitated. I sat down a safe distance from the bed, and he started to talk to me. "Aren't you the guy who lives in the van in the parking lot?" I said, "No, I live in Berkeley." He kept on talking about the guy in the van, but about every fifth sentence he'd say something like, "My stomach's really hurting." And then a few minutes of disconnected thoughts, and "I could use some milk," and more talk and, "Do we have any ice cream?" So I said, "Let me check," and there was ice cream. We ended up having an ice cream party together.
>
> What I've found in working with people with dementia, is that they require—almost in a visual sense—a softer focus that lets me tie one sentence in a paragraph to the related sentence in the next paragraph. I have to slow down enough to hear what this person's trying to communicate. I need to relax to hear that his stomach hurts and that he perceives that some kind of dairy product will make it feel better.
>
> I was there with him maybe a half hour altogether, and when I left I didn't think this guy was particularly demented any more. I don't think it was just me. I think he was clearer because I was able to hear him. Because he had been able to communicate.

It takes someone adept in active listening to do what Bharat does, to hear the thread of logic that runs through the seemingly incoherent ramblings of a person with dementia. But it's a learnable skill, as other caregivers can attest, based on compassion, attention, and the willingness to try.

✐ ✐ ✐ ✐

Bharat has particular compassion for people outside the mainstream, people who feel—or are made to feel—as if they "don't belong" because of race, sexual orientation, mental status, or other designations that are subordinate to the essential humanness of us all. In his work with people with AIDS, and in his work with other caregivers, Bharat has become a friend to many people from many different cultures, including various subcultures within the gay community. He has cared for men and women with histories of substance abuse and histories of prostitution, and with people of different races, nationalities, and belief systems. In all cases, he seeks to identify the individual's specific needs and circumstances.

I try to assess the client's needs as he or she defines them. For someone who's disenfranchised, without a home or medical insurance or income, maybe what she needs most is a place to live. For someone else, maybe they need to talk about their feelings before they can focus on filling out forms and taking care of business.

And with people who are especially difficult—provocative or hostile—I try not to be swept up in their projections of who they think I am, which involves checking if there's some truth to their projections. Am I being exclusive, or arrogant, or bigoted?

Sometimes it is the case that our differences are too great in the short amount of time we have to make contact. I may be available and ready, and the person in bed may not be.

Or he or she may be so fixed on my appearance as a blond, white male that the assumption is I can't possibly have anything to offer. At the same time, I have to keep developing my own nonjudgmentalness.

Sometimes cultural differences are the answers to what seemed unanswerable problems. A South African patient who consistently refused injections was labeled "uncooperative" by hospital residents until Bharat discovered that the man believed injections caused disease. He had been taught that during colonization, the British had injected black people with "medicines" that were supposed to do them good, but that in fact had spread terrible new diseases among them. He wasn't going to let it happen to him. Ultimately, the man was discharged from the hospital, but with more compassion and a lot less judgment than he would have been if Bharat hadn't probed for the source of his "refusal to cooperate."

When differences erupt between patient and health care providers, Bharat tries to remain his client's advocate. He steadfastly moves to facilitate dialogue between his clients and hospital personnel. He told me a story about a man who had been repotting a plant and been pricked by a thorn. People with HIV have to be especially careful of activities that put them in contact with harmful bacteria, which may be found in the garden, or in the manure in some potting soils, or living in the fish tank or bird cage or kitty litter box.

Bharat's client had had a badly compromised immune system, and within a matter of days his hand had become gangrenous. When he was admitted to San Francisco General, the surgery team wanted to amputate two fingers, but the man refused.

They put an incredible amount of pressure on him, and he still wouldn't do it, and finally, after several reevaluations, they realized that it was just the upper tissue of one finger that was necrotic. The hand, although it was quite scarred afterwards, healed fine with antibiotics and appropriate care.

In both these cases Bharat felt the best thing he could do was to support the client for having taken a courageous position and standing by it and following through. And in each case, the client was served because Bharat had listened to him and validated his right to his feelings.

> The greatest pain I've ever known has been of separation—
> that no one else has had the same feelings as me, and that
> I am somehow alone. When I've really gotten it that some-
> body else knew what I was feeling—that connection changes
> the experience of suffering. Stephen Levine [a much-respected
> teacher of hospice care] describes it as "transforming my pain
> into the pain." When you feel a collective awareness of the
> pain, it takes some of the weight off you, and it helps get you
> through the layers of separateness that usually exist between
> people.

"Getting through the layers of separateness," is how we get to what Bharat describes as a "cracking open":

> As much as I wish people didn't suffer, the fact is that often
> at the height of it something miraculous happens. I call it
> "cracking open." It's like a crevice appears in your everyday
> consciousness, and a light pours in through that crack.
> When that happens, I believe we get in touch with our
> essential nature.

Micaela Salort, whose story appears in this book, describes this same phenomenon as the "magic moment." Alex Martinez, another caregiver you'll meet in these pages, refers to it as the "encyclopedic moment." When it happens in the caregiving relationship, we resonate with our patient-partner like a tuning fork. Both the caregiver and the one cared for transcend their individual experience; neither is separate, neither is isolated, both are connected to a common center inside, a well of love and strength.

These experiences are characterized by a profound sense of unity with others. They can happen any time: when you are fully present to an anguished lover with AIDS, when you meet an old friend newly diagnosed with the HIV virus, or hold a newborn baby with AIDS, or your brother at the moment of his death. The feeling may come when you truly forgive someone, when you reunite. Or the feeling of deep connection may accompany vivid loving memories of friends and lovers who are gone. At such moments of grace we feel connected to a spiritual source, and that connection creates an environment in which fear moves to the background and the overriding feeling is one of profound unity with others.

Because of the client's more vulnerable circumstances, it is usually caregivers who make the first move to bridge the gap between themselves and their clients. To do so, the caregiver has to let go of some of his or her fears—of saying the wrong thing, of not being able to help.

One evening I was working late on the ward, and I walked by a room where there was a young black man I had only seen one other time in the dayroom in a wheelchair. He had declined very rapidly. He hadn't been out of his room for days and was believed close to death. It wasn't my intention to visit him—I was on my way to see another patient—but it was like I was sucked into the room.

He was clearly absolutely terrified. He had a bad case of AIDS-related pneumonia and he was hyperventilating. He was getting the maximum oxygen and humidifying air through this big mask with tubes coming out of it. It really amplifies the sound of the breath and it was a horrific image to see this young man lying there, his eyes like saucers, frozen in fear on a spot on the wall across from his bed. When I spoke to him, I knew he was there, but he couldn't take his eyes off that spot on the wall. He was so trying to maintain control that he was frozen. I leaned over into his gaze and put my hand on his chest lightly, and just stayed with him for a while, breathing with him, feeling totally lost about what to do. I had to help him, and I had to deal with my own anxiety because of my helplessness.

I've heard some people say sort of romantically that at a certain point of being with a dying person, that they gave that person permission to die. I think that concept is a way of taking care of yourself, reassuring yourself that it's okay.

I wanted to reassure him that it was okay. That was what kept coming up for me while I tried to figure out what to do in that situation. So I thought to tell him something about my own experience being around dying people. But I was new at the time, and I so much wanted to say the right thing, and be there, be the good counselor, and that really got in my way. I felt my role as caregiver slipping away and I knew I wasn't going to be any help to him, and finally I just told him where I was at.

I said, "It's really hard for me to see you so afraid like this, and I don't know what to say or do for you, but I can tell you something of what I've seen working with AIDS patients here. A lot of people report feeling a certain amount of equanimity and have had near-death experiences and described many things in common, and said that they realized they didn't have to be so afraid any more."

I just reported it, not even as a certainty. Just "This is what I've heard. . . ." This all took about fifteen minutes, and toward the end of that time his respirations started to slow and he started to calm down. He never moved his eyes, but I think I reassured him. I left and a few minutes later he died.

✸ ✸ ✸

Bharat is able to look into the eyes of a person in pain, of someone in terror, of someone who despairs, and not turn away. He perceives that he is looking through the window of the soul of the person he serves. Bharat is a devotee of the Hindu teacher Neem Karoli Baba, who some people believe is the incarnation of Hanuman, the mercurial monkey warrior in Hindu mythology.

> I resisted the idea of the guru. I was a confirmed atheist. But I've come to see that at a very basic level I'm inextricably connected with this certain spiritual lineage. I can't say I chose it—if I was to look at a menu, I wouldn't have chosen it. I was much more attracted to the Buddhist sensibility. But this teacher in my life is an archetypal form through which I see the divine. He is the form of the divine that I relate to.
> Hanuman was a great warrior and a demi-God who served his beloved Lord Rama with boundless enthusiasm. So he's an example for me. My spiritual work is about service. And service has many forms, whether it's bringing someone a video, or an ice cream, or changing soiled linens. The more I make contact through the eyes, the more I know how to serve. It's all, "I am giving to you because I love you so much. I'm trying to find you in there. And I want to somehow serve you."

Bharat's service is his doorway to the realm of shared awareness and the experience of his essential nature. He says that his practices, such as meditation, or the repetition of his mantra, or use of prayer beads, or chanting, or even sometimes exercising, help keep him primed for that consciousness and that experience.

> I find the more I'm in myself the more impact I can have by developing what's been called "a healing presence." Basically, I try to see the person I'm sitting with. When I'm really clear, when I look into his eyes, even though that person might be hard to look at because the disease has ravaged him, I know that it's only my guru in a distressing disguise looking back at me, sometimes laughing at me because I thought it was someone else.

When Bharat looks into the eyes of his clients with AIDS and sees his guru, he sees the eternal in them, he sees what he calls the divine, just as Mother Teresa sees Christ in her lepers in Calcutta. And when Bharat looks into the eyes of his patients with AIDS and opens his heart to their divinity, he is *with them*. He is touched by divinity too. "When that happens," he told me, "I'm much less caught in the drama of everything, the suffering, the tragedy, the loss." I asked him, "Is that like the connection the wounded healer makes—the one that transcends the drama?"

Yes, but I resist romanticizing the wounded healer, as I've seen done in some psychological communities—as if some people are wounded and some aren't. I think to be born is to be wounded. We all suffer from that primary separation. That's the root wound, as I understand it. And sharing that, that's when we come together.

Do you tell your clients that you're HIV positive?

I don't usually. But if it's clear we have a limited amount of time and if I think it will help me bridge faster with another person, I might tell him or tell her that I've been positive too, for nine years. It does seem to open up a lot of possibilities for the other person. I don't know if it's true, but I believe it is, that they see me as more understanding, knowing what it's like—the fearful nights, certain kinds of dreams, the social stigma, and how it all erodes our self-esteem if we internalize it.

You sound as if you have some experience internalizing it.

Oh, I've had moments of feeling like I was sewage. I've seen myself as some kind of deviant. There's a real propensity to feel very guilty that it's happened, that you should never have sex again, that you're polluted, toxic. You wonder if you really deserve a certain quality of care, or the respect of the people who treat you.

Some people with AIDS and some HIV+ caregivers can be fiercely self-critical, having internalized the shaming voices of the family and society. The loneliness, fear, anger, or depression that those voices inspire is what we refer to as psychological pain.

━ ━ ━ ━

The caregiver, especially at the end of a client's life, can be drawn into that person's inner world, where spirit and psyche reside. Some of Bharat's most insightful comments about caregiving have to do with his deep understanding of the distinctions and connections between one's belief system and his or her unique psychological history.

The psychological and the spiritual are very connected for me. When I'm in a room with someone, I'm often balancing between the two.

Some people have their spiritual philosophy down pat, but they're totally in denial about their unfinished psychological business. They've got a lot of grief, but they smile through their teeth and say, "Isn't the dying process rich?" Then there are people who get totally lost in the emotional pain and lose the spiritual perspective.

I try to use methods from both disciplines. For example, if I have an aversion to someone, I can process my emotions even while I'm sitting with that person, and realize maybe that this person reminds me of my father. And tell myself, "This is not my father; this is my own unfinished business." And then I can bring myself back to the moment with the person.

A lot of people in the spiritual community have tried to skip over their personal work, and come crashing down. The problem is in regulating how much we process the psychological. I think you can overdo it, examining your emotions, your history, your personal story over and over again.

I'm also aware that my personal attachment to the spiritual sometimes makes me insensitive. That was especially so when I first started doing AIDS work. I came from a middle-class Anglo perspective into the room of a person of color, or some disenfranchised person, thinking, "God, you're really stuck in this suffering. If you would just do these spiritual practices I can show you, you'll see the truth." I really didn't get at all what it's like to be someone who lives on the street, or an addict, or a person with no friends. I feel more solid now in terms of being sensitive, and also in terms of endurance. I feel like I surf those tidal waves in the charting room a little better these days.

✦ ✦ ✦

Bharat told me that he used to have a "romantic notion of what it was like to counsel people with AIDS, but that has fallen away." Now he knows that "compassion isn't necessarily all hugs and the usual show of affection. I think sometimes it's very fierce."

His words remind me of those of the poet Rainer Maria Rilke, who wrote to a patroness during his final excruciating illness: "Whoever does not, sometime or other, give his full consent, his full and joyous consent to the dreadfulness of life, can never take possession of the unutterable abundance and power of our existence."[1]

You hear about heroic efforts that caregivers make on their clients' behalf, and that people with AIDS make to survive, but fighting for life is human nature, and laying one's hand on the chest of a dying man to comfort him is a humble enough gesture. It is the Wounded Healer who embodies an alternative to the Hero among AIDS caregivers and the people they serve. Instead of the Hero's penchant for combat and conquest, the Healer seeks connection and understanding, and many of our caregivers find these through psychospiritual learning, exploration, and growth. Bharat's teachers, mentors, and spiritual advisers, and the support of friends and colleagues, are central to his work and his way of life—unlike the heroic individualist who is reluctant to ask for help.

In fact, caregivers help best through partnership with clients, which is the essence of the Wounded Healer's practice.

- - - -

Bharat doesn't try to conquer pain or suffering. He goes into the darkness with his clients, at some risk to his own well-being, given his HIV status. He enters a place with them where there is fear, confusion, inadequacy, anger, and despair, but where there is also the possibility of resolving personal conflicts and inner chaos, and sometimes achieving transformation. This place exists both within and beyond the ego, and in it resides the source for our deepest healing, a source called variously God, or Spirit, or the Source of Life, to name a few of its thousand appellations.

Note

1. From a letter to Countess Crouy, April 1923.

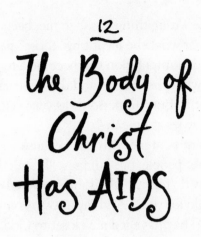

12
The Body of Christ Has AIDS

I know there's a broken piece in me, a wounded part. It took me a long time to make friends with that, and I will never deny it about myself again.

Jacinta helps make a home for people with AIDS at the Center for AIDS Services in Oakland, California. Here men and women with AIDS find a welcoming environment, a meal, counseling, a place to wash their clothes. For many it is the first home, the first safe haven, that they have had in a very long time. Jacinta is a Roman Catholic nun—has been for more than forty years—and she says that during her AIDS ministry these past six years, she has come to experience God more deeply than ever before.

I've been told more than once that I'm a disappointment as a Roman Catholic nun. I'd been in the AIDS ministry perhaps a year, when one of the sisters who is part of my community said to me, in an unfriendly tone of voice, "What do you do for those people?"

It's just the wrong thing to say to me, because I bristle all over. I asked her what she meant by "those" people. Sometimes this kind of interaction can become a teaching. It causes people to say what they mean, and then you can have a dialogue about it. But this person was very defensive. She said, "You know what I mean."

I didn't want to argue with her, because we were at a table with other people, but I did say, "I don't do anything for them. They do for me." And she answered, "What could they possibly do for you?" And my answer is my deepest belief. I said, "They have led me closer to God."

In fact, when I went into AIDS ministry it was like coming home. I saw these people who had to face their own woundedness—and not just one person, but many people— and when I saw that, I found the courage to look inside and face my own. I've wandered around so long looking for a home, and all the time home was inside.

*　*　*

Jacinta's path to home and God has been a difficult one, made more so because of a feeling of inferiority—the result of a neurological disability she suffered from childhood on, which was not diagnosed until she was an adult.

If my brain tells my hands to do something, they may or may not do it, or they may do something else, or they may not do it now. My brain doesn't coordinate well with my hands. When I'm writing, too, my hand won't always put the letters I need on the page; sometimes it will write something different.

I had a handicap. But I didn't know it was a handicap, and no one acknowledged it as such. Instead, I thought I just couldn't do anything right. Accomplishing what I thought other people expected me to seemed the most important thing. But early on they put me out of gym classes, and then they took me out of dancing. And everything I got taken out of made me surer that I wasn't a good person, and that no one could ever love me.

Even when I entered the religious community, this certainty persisted. I could handle the study part fine, but the other things they expected me to do, play the organ, sew, drive a car—I couldn't do any of these things, so I was left out of them. I felt excluded. And more and more I began to feel as if I just didn't count.

It was when I was trying to learn how to drive that the instructor said to me, "Your hands don't follow what you tell them to do too well." It was the first time anyone had suggested there was something wrong. I was forty years old.

Jacinta persevered as a nun, taking on as much responsibility as she could in areas where she was not handicapped, to balance what she considered to be her shortcomings. By 1974 she was a superior at one of her order's houses in Southern California. Her responsibilities included teaching at the local seminary, supervising three other sisters and their parishes, and directing an educational program for two thousand children.

It was too much. Jacinta experienced what she refers to as a "break." It seemed to have broken her at the time, but it turned out to be just the break she needed. She admitted to her mother superior that she couldn't handle the weight of her job, and she was relieved of her position.

I felt so ashamed in the community because I was the first sister ever taken out of office. I really felt worthless. But that break forced me into therapy, individual and group.

Group therapy was the first experience I ever had of saying who I really was. And it gave me the opportunity to talk about the fact that I had been molested as a child, which my

family never knew, and which had enhanced my believing
I wasn't worth anything.

I imagine how Jacinta must have felt as a child. She had been
abused by a family acquaintance, which must have shaken her trust
in people; she had a neurological problem that made her feel out of
control of her physical body and certainly shook her trust in herself.
But in spite of feelings of unworthiness, she believed that God
called her to serve, and she put her faith in that, and dedicated herself to Him.

Loving God didn't erase past injuries, though. What *does* work
to make things right and make Jacinta feel better about herself is
the love and acceptance she shares with those people who come to
the Center—in spite of the fact that some of these people may be
suspicious of her, or feel that talking to a nun implies a moral fail-
ing on their part, or that accepting her kind of support is another
blow to self-esteem. These are people who are frequently unwilling
to examine or even admit to unpleasant things about themselves.

Jacinta's ministry works for those she serves because she identifies with the disenfranchised people who feel bad in the same ways
she has, who feel alienated from God because they feel worthless in
other people's eyes. It works because, having made the transition
herself, she knows how to help them experience God's love. It
works because she sees their value as human beings, and reflects it
back to them so that they can see it too.

There's a piece of me that feels their pain. It's not something
I learned anywhere; it's something I live. They may be suffering for a different reason than me, but pain has a similar ring
to it. You recognize it.

I recognized it in Hakeem, who came to the Center about
a year ago. I had great respect for him, but I was also afraid
of him. I knew he was a tough customer.

As Hakeem and I got acquainted, I began to admire a
very honest streak in him. One time he told us that we some-

times put people in compromising positions by asking them
to help out in areas where they can't but be tempted to steal.
He said he'd appreciate it if we would get more tuned into
that. I liked Hakeem's honesty. I know that the people I care
for are the key to my becoming a better caregiver. I have to
be willing sometimes to hear that what I'm saying is wrong,
or what I'm doing is wrong, and I have to find out why. So
I told Hakeem that I appreciated his telling me this, and we
began to get closer.

Then he got very ill and it seemed like he was dying. He
went to the hospital, and it was when I visited him there that
he told me he had murdered three people.

He had done twenty years in prison. He had done his
time, but he needed to know that God forgave him. It was
a very touching moment when he told me this. I also used
to think that God couldn't love me because of all the things
I'd done wrong. I'd spent so much of my life thinking I had
to "be good" to please God, or that something I did would
upset God. But that's not the God I know now, not the real
God that I have a very personal relationship with. How
wrong it would be to look at Hakeem and think that God
didn't love him!

I didn't have to talk religion with Hakeem. I knew I just
needed to hold him and God would let him know He loved
him. So we prayed a little, and cried together, and then
Hakeem got very quiet, and he smiled and said "Thank you.
I know now that that's all squared away."

Jacinta has learned from her experience at the Center, as many
caregivers do from their clients, that personal tragedy can be a turning point, that it can create unexpected alliances. It can also focus
one on the deep personal questions: Who am I? How do I relate to
life (and death) around me? What are my values? For many caregivers, as for many people with AIDS, an intimacy with suffering is
the beginning of heightened psychological and spiritual awareness.

▰ ▰ ▰

Taking the journey from the church to the Center was an act of extraordinary courage for Jacinta. She is devoted to Catholicism. Her faith is strong. But she faced the possibility of the same kind of rejection that the church has dealt many of the people who use the Center, when she took her first steps in that direction. She knew that unless she could develop a healthy autonomous sense of herself both apart from and in relation to her church, she would be forever imprisoned by certain of its attitudes that she could not share.

Jacinta embarked on her journey not knowing who she was or what she wanted. She realized that she might never know unless she wandered, took risks, and transformed an identity based on her role as a religious person, into one based on psychological and spiritual questions about herself in relation to the world. The journey was to be one of self-discovery.

She would stay true to her understanding of Christlike compassion, and in the course of her new ministry would adopt another tenet—that of unconditional love, both given and received. Today Jacinta is still a devoted follower of Christ, with a humanist vision:

> I think the whole idea of following Christ means finding Christ in people in the street. If we were there when Christ walked this earth, we would have found him there. Have you seen the button that says, THE BODY OF CHRIST HAS AIDS? If we believed that, if we saw that the people in the street with AIDS are Christ, then we'd treat them as we would treat Christ. I meet Him regularly this way.

In stepping into the streets, carrying with her both love and compassion, opening her heart to the people she cares for, and largely leaving judgmental attitudes behind, Jacinta makes a difference in the world and in herself. This diminutive woman with the sweet smile has forged deep emotional connections with others who have known the feeling of inadequacy, of difference, of rejection, and lack of love. In becoming comfortable with a new feisty self, who was able to speak out on behalf of others and herself, Jacinta also became comfortable with her tough and streetwise clients, and their right to speak out. She says that when she is with people who occupy the margins of mainstream society, people very unlike any she had known in sixty years of living, she can be more herself than with anyone else.

◢ ◢ ◢

Chris was one of my first teachers at the Center. I was new here and feeling like I didn't know anything. He was a pagan. As we got to know each other, I understood that he had been searching for truth. He had been into satanic worship and witchcraft and some pretty rough stuff. I had never known anyone like that—all that inside one little human being! He used to say, "We're a funny combination." We were.

Chris was the first person I had met who was very ill and dying that I couldn't—or didn't feel I should—use the word God with. It was like my God prop was gone and now what do I do? Once he even asked me, "Aren't you supposed to tell me that if I don't believe in God, when I die I'll go to hell?" And I said, "No way am I supposed to do that," because I knew it wasn't true.

He was trying to push me to preach at him because that was what he thought Catholic nuns did. I didn't fill the role for him. And he certainly wasn't what I understood a pagan to be. Our relationship became very intimate because we eventually let each other *be* without any roles. And that was scary, although it was something we both longed for, because we both knew we were deeper than the roles other people had created for us.

As Jacinta becomes more herself and less her role, she begins to demonstrate some of the "in your face" courage her clients have taught her: "I can say now for the first time in my life that I have

courage. I have the courage to be me, which is what I feared most."
She tells a story that exemplifies her courage:

> Michael had come into the Center feeling so bad that we
> took him to the doctor, and when the doctor saw him she
> put him right in the hospital. He had left his little apartment
> in a bad neighborhood in Berkeley "unsecured." Someone
> would have to go over there and lock the windows. I asked
> one of the other staff members, Tom, to come with me.
>
> When we got to the apartment, I could hear sounds from
> inside. We were scared to death, but we knocked on the door.
> This big guy answered. There were two men, two women,
> and seven children who had moved into Michael's apartment.
> He had only been gone one day.
>
> I told them, "This isn't your apartment. You have to
> leave." The big man said, "We can't leave. We've got little
> children here." I told him I was there to secure the apartment,
> and I intended to do it, and he had to leave. He asked for just
> one hour, and I said, "I'm not giving you any time at all.
> You have to leave now."
>
> We went inside, and I don't know whether it was con-
> sciously or not that we backed ourselves into the kitchen and
> up against the kitchen drawers. My thought was, if there's any-
> thing in here that can be a weapon it's going to be in these
> drawers.
>
> The man got really nasty, but they started moving their
> things out. He said to Tom, "She has no right to wear that
> cross, she doesn't love God at all. She doesn't even care about
> these little children." He knew just how to get to me. And he
> said, "She's nothing but a fucking momma." It was one of
> those things I couldn't take too personally.
>
> This was something I had to do for Michael, but it was
> hard for me to see the children go. But I've had to come to
> grips with the fact that I'm not here to save the world. My

clients come first to me. Michael came above all four of those adults and all those children.

They had come in through the window. That's the way of the streets. An apartment is vacant—they knew he was sick because they asked me how sick he was. We finally got them to leave. Michael returned home not too much later.

＊＊＊

Jacinta continues to discover herself through her AIDS ministry. She says that profound learning is occurring in the midst of AIDS-related destruction. What she has learned has deepened her vision and her purpose and her faith in herself and her God. She has learned much about humanity in her service, but also much about inhumanity:

> January 12 is the anniversary of Leo's death. Leo died as a result of a gay bashing. For me it was the most devastating thing that's ever happened—seeing what one human can do to another. And then try to work through forgiveness for those that did it. Leo could. He somehow had the grace, he had the gift. I was almost angry with him because he was so forgiving.
>
> I didn't get over Leo's death. I buried my feelings, but later I had to take two weeks' leave of absence. That's never happened to me before. It was my horror at the brutality of people, and at not being able to forgive.

Leo's death was gruesome, but HIV can sometimes seem as cruel. Caregivers on the front lines of the AIDS pandemic may experience moments of horror at the brutality and senselessness of the disease, and at the lack of justice that seems a part of it. You begin to ask questions when you're living with AIDS, even if you're not HIV positive. And death is something you question. Death is something you think about a lot.

Jacinta told me about two men from the Center who died recently:

> They chose to use street drugs until it just did them in. That's
> the way they died. But what could anyone do? As a caregiver,
> I know I need to let my clients express their feelings. I need
> to let them be just where they are.
> But it's the hardest thing for me. I hate that they use
> their money for drugs and that they steal from us for drugs.
> I let them come back day after day. I still care about them,
> but it's hard. I have to separate them from their behavior.
> I have to acknowledge that I don't know what it's like to be
> on drugs or to have a life in which drugs make sense.

This is genuine acceptance and unconditional love, the essential lesson of all religions, and precisely what Jacinta wants and needs for herself. Her acceptance and love are also her strongest allies in her work with people with AIDS—along with the knowledge that she can't help everyone who comes to the Center. Though it saddens her, she doesn't blame herself for other people's self-destructive behavior. Less experienced caregivers frequently do and may be crushed by not being able to "save" their clients.

✦✦✦✦

Dealing with the death of a client is often a part of the caregiving experience. For most caregivers, this is a very difficult part of the work. It has been so for Jacinta.

> Chris taught me something about death. He used to say,
> "I'm not afraid to die, I just don't want to be there when it
> happens." But one time we talked seriously about it and he
> said he really wasn't afraid. He said, "I've never been peaceful. And now I'm getting peaceful. I'm getting very close to
> death." He equated peace and death.

At our last meeting Chris taught me about respect. He told me he wanted me to take a vacation from him. I didn't know what he meant. He said, "I want you to tell me good-bye today, to say what we need to each other today, and I don't want you to come back to see me anymore."

He said that I had been there when he had needed me most and when he had been most himself, and now they would begin to increase his morphine, and he wouldn't be himself in some ways, and he didn't want me to see that.

I said, "Okay," I could accept what he said. But I did not want this to be my last time to see Chris. I wanted to be with him when he was dying, and he was cutting me out of that. I knew our relationship was strong enough that I didn't have to be with him, but I wanted to. I also knew it was important not to put my agenda onto him, but I wanted to.

Then, before I left, Chris said to me, "You know, in ten or twelve years you're going to join me and we'll be together forever in the hereafter."

That really touched me very deeply, because I knew then that Chris had met God, or whatever word we use for the higher being or greater power, and what he was saying was true. I kissed him goodbye, and as I was leaving the room, he called my name. When I turned, he said, "You know, it might even be less than ten or twelve years."

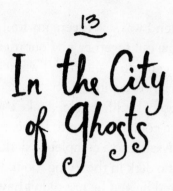

13

In the City of Ghosts

George Simmons is another veteran of the AIDS front lines, having served as a Shanti caregiver since the mid-1980s. Today he is one of Shanti's four volunteer coordinators, and brings a wealth of hard-won wisdom to his work.

> I think that caregiving is a great opportunity to discover that you can be of incredible service and benefit to another person. But I would give it all up—everything I've learned in the last ten years—for AIDS to never have happened.
>
> It's changed me. A lot of people have become more spiritual caring for people with AIDS. I've become less so. I don't look at caregiving as some spiritual journey. It's too painful, and too many people suffer. Not to say that I don't have beliefs. But this is simply an enormous tragedy. I don't believe in any kind of God that would let this happen. I'm more of a realist.

George's realism and down-to-earth qualities are critical components of his caregiving skills. But George can also be intuitive and attentive, as this story about his friend Raoul demonstrates:

I met Raoul when I was seventeen, my freshman year in college. We came out together, and our friendship was one of the reasons I came to California. I was really shocked when he was diagnosed with AIDS.

Near the end of his life I helped take care of him. I had a key because he couldn't get up to let people in anymore. One day I let myself into a completely dark house and found him sitting in the dark in the living room. I asked him what he was doing, and he said he just didn't have the energy to get up and turn the lights on.

But I thought there was more to it than that. So I quietly walked through the house and turned on all the lights except in the living room. And then I went back and sat down with him. I didn't say anything, but after a short time he told me that he was sitting in the dark because he wanted to see what it was going to be like.

I know if I had rushed around and turned on all the lights, he would never have told me this. He had CMV and he was especially fearful about going blind. It was one of the big quality-of-life issues that he talked about. He was a very visual person. He had been a gardener and a florist.

He was incredibly depressed and he was letting go. He's one of the few people I've seen on a daily basis who really grieved the fact of his dying. The dark represented his loss of vision as well as his losing his life. He had already lost his mobility, his ability to work, which he had loved, and a lot of friends who abandoned him because he was sick. He had lost almost everything by the time he died.

When he was in the hospital for the last time, I took a day off to be with him. When I arrived he was very anxious. He confided to me that he was planning to tell his doctor that he didn't want any more treatment—except for his CMV meds. That told me that even though he was giving up, he didn't want to give up completely.

We talked about it. I wasn't going to argue with him, he knew that. And I knew that giving him permission to talk or cry or ask questions would help relieve his anxiety. You realize that the person probably does have a pretty good intuitive sense of what he wants, and that your role is just to help him see that.

I asked him if he was frightened, and he said he was only afraid that stopping his treatments, he might be in pain. He took prophylaxis for pneumocystis, and something for his neuropathy, and all these other drugs they give people with AIDS.

It wasn't easy for him to talk about this, not even to me, and we were close. With the doctor, it was really hard. When he finally got out that he wanted to stop the meds, the doctor said, "Do you understand what this means?" and Raoul said, "Yes."

But then he couldn't say what else was on his mind. He stammered and stuttered, and I saw he couldn't get around his fear to ask the question he most wanted to know, so finally I did. I said, "Will he be in any pain?" and the doctor said, "No, of course not. We'll make sure that you're not in pain."

Raoul and I spent six more hours together that day, and they were the best hours that we had had with one another in years—reminiscing. Raoul talking about life, what it had meant, his regrets. It was an incredibly beautiful, sad day. Afterward, I understood that we would never have had that day together if I had not somehow given him permission to tell me what he wanted. I don't think he would have been able to tell his doctor what he wanted without having told me first.

When a person with AIDS grapples with the difficult question of whether or when to discontinue treatment, the advocacy of someone who cares is especially valuable. The subject is fraught with the tacit acknowledgment of death's inevitability. It is full of the unknown. In Raoul's case, would his doctor support his decision, would he be able to manage the pain, would he be—even unconsciously—disappointed in Raoul for "defecting," and move on to other, more "hopeful" cases?

Confronting this issue often pulls the person with AIDS, as well as the family, friends, and caregivers close to him or her, into a vortex of grief over the loss being contemplated. For some people, making the choice is difficult enough. The added burden of communicating their choice, especially to physicians or to loved ones who may not be willing or ready to hear it, can be excruciating. The presence of an advocate and spokesperson may be vital.

For George, there is no particular protocol in the service of his clients, other than paying attention, reaffirming commitment, and being an advocate, when necessary. These are the characteristics of the client advocate: he doesn't criticize or judge his client's choices, but he is ready to talk about them, to help the anxious client examine options. Although he is ready to help, he is careful to keep his own agenda, feelings, and desires secondary, and put his client's up front. He cedes control to the client. He stands by. He is receptive, not overly directive, helping his client find his own way to his own conclusion. He does not direct or interfere with the content of his client's conversation or discussion with health professionals or loved ones.

✒ ✒ ✒

George was four or five when his parents went through an acrimonious divorce. He and his sister were raised by his paternal grandparents in Indiana; they didn't see their mother again until George was an adolescent. One of the children's aunts became their surrogate mother, and her death from cancer when George was in his twenties was especially painful. So loss is something George knows about from way back, and working in the AIDS community for the past decade has magnified the experience.

For me, San Francisco is a city of ghosts. I see them on the streets. Somebody comes around the corner, and I go, "Oh, wow, there's Mark!" Well, it isn't Mark because Mark is dead. But there's that momentary glimpse, that moment when you really want it to be Mark. And then you have to go through the emotional stuff of its not being Mark.

It's a very bittersweet place, San Francisco, just because of the enormity of the loss. More so for me, maybe, because of my job. The number of people with AIDS whom I've known—friends, volunteers, clients—to catalogue all those losses is pretty incredible.

People disappear here. They die, they're cremated, and they're gone. It adds a very surreal aspect to AIDS. Where I grew up, when people die, they lie in a funeral home for three days and you see them, and you go to the cemetery and see them buried. It may sound morbid, but these are very valuable rituals. In San Francisco there are all these ethereal people floating around because I've never seen them dead. I have seen some people dead—but then there are all these other people who are just gone.

Are George's ghosts a destructive fantasy? Psychopathology? Not at all; in fact, such glimpses are a common experience for care-givers, especially for those who have experienced the deaths of many clients and friends and lovers, and whose losses number in the dozens or even hundreds. With such numbers, it is very difficult to "process" or "work through" each and every death as we might under other circumstances. It can't be done in an instant, and psy-chologically speaking, the bodies begin to pile up. Without that "coming to terms with," it is hard for us to put our dead to rest.

The disappearances that George speaks of represent the ulti-mate in lack of closure and are especially disturbing to him because they resonate with the disappearance of his mother and his beloved aunt, and the feeling of unfinished business he experiences over them. It's the same for all of us, when those close to us disappear physically or emotionally and we haven't had the chance to settle our accounts with them.

✦ ✦ ✦ ✦

I had a good friend with AIDS who had been having symptoms of mild dementia. I had been away at a weeklong conference, and when I returned I couldn't reach him by phone. I went over to his apartment and found him dead. He had taken his life. He had been dead several days. It really was the most devastating death I've experienced, including my father's, because Joel was an incredibly kind, gentle, sweet man. And the way he died—I couldn't get over it being a suicide. That he died alone. That he'd been dead in his apartment for days. The whole thing was horrific. I felt, if life can do this to him, what's it going to do to the rest of us? I was a mess for about three months. I just went into shock and came to work—I was trying to do my job at the time—I think I got three days bereavement leave or something.

I've had years now to process Joel's death, but I still feel he didn't deserve to die that way. I've learned from it, though. I've learned that I can withstand practically any shock, and operate under pretty difficult circumstances.

With every shock withstood, and every difficult circumstance confronted, George feels that he gets stronger—perhaps proving Nietzsche's optimistic adage, "Anything that does not kill me makes me stronger."

For caregivers in San Francisco these past dozen years, enormous strength has been necessary for survival, not only to do what they can for their clients or friends, but to withstand the realization of what they *can't* do for them. For many, AIDS is in some ways a test of endurance. Caregivers like George, who were forced to find their own resources for survival from an early age because they couldn't count on parents for it, may be especially durable.

IN THE CITY OF GHOSTS   173

Their adversity has made them strong enough to discover a dear friend's decomposing body, to witness a best friend's grief, to walk among ghosts.

Surviving in the high-frequency, high-tension, high-wire act that is the world of AIDS means understanding the nature of life as tenuous at best. You develop the psychology of a survivor, adapting to the dynamic interplay of physical, psychological, social, and spiritual factors, to serve in these times of extremity. You feel a kinship with others who endure and survive. You live in a state that is different from a crisis with a definable beginning, middle, and end. Your situation is ongoing, and you are aware that this will probably remain the circumstance for the rest of your client's life, and perhaps your own. You learn an attitude—if you are a survivor, you say, as George does: "I think people need to acknowledge that this thing is going to be around for a long time, and that in spite of it you can still have a good life."

I experience the pain. But I don't think it's possible to do this work well if you don't let it go. If I left Shanti every day with just a fraction of what I've heard, I couldn't function under the emotional assault of it all because when I leave here I go home and deal with friends who are seropositive, who are symptomatic. I'm always aware when I'm with them that I better enjoy them now, because they won't be around later.

But there are times that I want to get on a plane and get as far away from here as I can. I'm sad and a mess for a couple of days, and then I'm better. I don't try to run away from the feelings anymore. Once I was in one of these moods, and my friend said, "You know, George, if you go you'll be taking your mind with you." I told him it was a risk I was willing to take.

In one sense, survival in the AIDS era is a kind of debt we pay to those who have died. In surviving ourselves, we allow our dead brothers and sisters, friends and lovers, to live on in us. In sharing their stories, we let them live on in the world. They become reminders and representatives of our collective struggle, part of our experience, helping shape our evolving identities. This incorporation of the dead within one's psyche and one's world is anything but a neurotic pattern. It is part of how the survivor attempts to heal himself and continue caring in a city of ghosts.

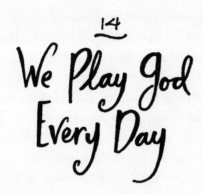

14
We Play God Every Day

It's a double-edged sword: what my strength is in private practice is also what tears me apart. I do get involved, and I probably break a lot of the rules in terms of the doctor-patient
relationship, but it's also why I'm considered good at what I do,
because I put myself into it.

Tom Schiller is a physician who specializes in treating people
with AIDS. Tom is a dream doctor. He listens. I mean he *really*
listens. He is aware of the effect of AIDS on one's body and mind,
and he addresses both in his efforts to heal. As far as he's concerned,
standard rules governing a doctor's approach to his or her patients
don't always apply with this particular disease.

Tom counts among his resources "the doctor within the
patient," as the great philosopher-physician Albert Schweitzer
called it: the patient's own expertise, intelligence, and will. Tom
rejects the idea of the passive patient who suffers silently through
endless tests, medications, and interventions. He believes the "let
the doctor do it" approach strips the patient of incentive and
responsibility. When a patient leaves his decisions to his physician,

he surrenders some of his personal resources, some of his fight for survival and some of the ability to heal himself. The physician who encourages this kind of abdication, sends the message that personal resources and the doctor-patient relationship are insignificant factors in the practice of medicine. Tom says quite the opposite.

Larry Hjort, whose story appears in an earlier chapter, is one of Tom Schiller's patients. When I said to Tom that Larry certainly didn't subscribe to the "let the doctor do it" approach, he laughed. Larry had interviewed several doctors before settling on him. Tom understood and even welcomed Larry's desire to be involved, to disagree, to get second opinions, to compare notes with friends.

> I wish I had more patients like Larry. He's assertive because he's got a lot on the line. He wants as much control over his destiny as he can have. Yet for as many Larrys as there are, there are just as many who won't participate at all. Then the burden is all on me, and I'd just as soon not carry it alone.
>
> A doctor has to be willing to give up some of the control he's used to having. But on the patient's side, if he's too demanding, he'll burn everyone out.

Striking the right balance, sharing the burden, allows patients like Larry to become part of the decision-making process, and therefore part of the healing process. But what Larry and Tom have by way of a partnership in Larry's health care is unusual. Often the patient and the doctor represent two sides instead of a united front, which handicaps their relationship from the start. Too often, the doctor-patient relationship is strained and unpleasant. Some patients consider doctors guilty until proven otherwise, based on previous experiences with physicians or other authority figures.

Dealing with this kind of anger and suspicion is tough on the doctor. Tom makes a preemptive move toward cooperation and mutual respect by demonstrating his genuine interest in his patient's needs and preferences, by both his willingness to listen to his patient's story and his desire for consensus on how they will proceed to treat the disease.

The assurance that I give my patients—that I'll carry out their wishes concerning terminal care, even if that differs from the family's or significant other's preference—generally makes me a confidant as well. I often get privileged information that helps us enhance the patient's overall care that wouldn't have been shared with me otherwise.

I learned as a resident on the cancer ward that when the inevitable approaches it's critical to spend a few extra minutes with the patient and to listen to what he or she is telling you, whether by metaphor, or through body language. The challenge is not to figure out what treatment will buy them a few more days, but to discover what you can do to help them reach a comfort level, or peace with dying, and to reassure them that you'll help them be comfortable.

* * * *

A good doctor-patient relationship begins with a painstaking, unhurried history that will serve as a model for future dialogues in which the doctor will listen carefully for what is said and what is unsaid.

I wish they taught medical students that when you take a history you may ask the same questions every time, but you'll have to ask them differently for every patient. Most doctors approach every patient the same way. They approach the disease, not the patient. They have a checklist, but they don't hear about the bad headaches or some chronic symptom because they don't take the time to let the person say what else is going on.

The tendency is for the doctor to ask closed rather than open questions of the patient to collect the history: "Have you experienced night sweats?" "Have you had any fevers?" Rather than, "Tell me how you've been feeling." The latter takes longer, but the former misses too much.

Unfortunately, an economic fact of life for many physicians is that history taking is not a money-making activity, as many other procedures are. The younger, often debt-ridden physician, or the older, financially over-committed one, may focus on activities that maximize income. This approach does not include questions about the patient's emotional or social life. It does not necessitate attention to nonverbal communication. These doctors don't listen for faltering speech, or watch for a diverted gaze or nervous tic that suggests something troublesome and unspoken.

If it's appropriate, Tom will let a patient know that they have something in common. Tom is gay. He lives in the same community as many of his patients, has known self-denigration, and the search for acceptance—both self-acceptance and the acceptance of others.

"If the patient knows you understand, it's easier to talk to you, easier to trust you," Tom says. "If you let that little bit of yourself out there, you'll probably get a whole lot back."

This is not to say, necessarily, that straight doctors are at a disadvantage establishing an empathic relationship with their gay HIV-positive patients. It does mean that many straight doctors have much to learn about gay and lesbian couples. They may not know how to interact with a patient's lover, or not allow him or her access to information about a patient that they would a spouse or parent. Every doctor who works with people with AIDS and accepts his or her patient's situation, a gay lifestyle, IV drug use—whatever it is—can learn to establish an empathic and healing relationship with that patient. But discriminatory or prejudicial attitudes, whether conscious or not, can be insidious and injurious to people who are already dealing with the pain of AIDS. Racism, sexism, homophobia, and judgmental attitudes toward IV drug users are forms of violence. Leveled by a doctor against a vulnerable patient, they are particularly abhorrent. But such assaults occur too frequently in many places.

I've had airline stewards fly in once a month from Salt Lake City or Minnesota because they couldn't get care in their own city, or the response was, you have that diagnosis, you're dead. One patient had three or four hundred T-cells. He needed a simple hernia repair. He had to come to San Francisco to have it done.

When one of my first patients was dying, his mother who ran a little nursing home facility back in Arkansas with five or six residents came and got him and took him back home to care for him. And she couldn't get care for him back there. They threatened to take away her license because her son was living in her home. But she was stoic. She dealt with it. She still sends me Christmas cards.

～～～

What happens when a person's health is miserable and will never substantially improve, when he or she is extremely uncomfortable due to a number of bodily failures, or when the pain can't be managed well, and radical incontinence and diarrhea are daily occurrences? What happens when the patient says he has nothing to live for because all his close friends have died of AIDS? What if he says that death will be a release, and you know he's probably right? For many people with AIDS, there comes a time when they must consider whether to continue trying to prolong their life, or whether to "let go," by which we mean refusing any more aggressive treatment in the direction of physical improvement. Imagine how it would be to confront this decision alone, without a knowledgeable friend to help you make an informed choice, or acknowledge the gravity of the decision, or honor the choice you make. And yet, Tom maintains that many doctors will not be that knowledgeable friend. "Some doctors fall back on the Hippocratic oath as their reason for not dealing with death and dying," Tom told me. "I call it the hypocritical oath. They say, 'We can't play God.' We play God every day!"

Every time we resuscitate a patient, feed them intravenously for prolonged periods, or keep them on a ventilator chronically, we play God. I'll do everything I can to keep a patient alive who has quality time left, which only the individual patient can truly decide.

When I can no longer help my patients achieve quality of life, my focus becomes their suffering, and their need for choice and dignity as they face death. I think it's unethical to continue unwanted and futile treatments, or to pressure patients to do so—although it's often the easier course, especially if the family wants it.

Frank was Tom's lover who died of AIDS two years ago. Tom talked about how they handled Frank's wanting to "let go."

Frank didn't want to let anyone down. I told him it was his life. His friends weren't nauseated twenty-four hours a day. They didn't have diarrhea twenty times a day. But I called all the people he talked about letting down, and told them he needed to hear it from them. I said, "There's no more time for rah-rah. That's not the support he needs now. Now he needs to know that even though you don't want to lose him, you understand that he's had enough." And everyone did. This not only let Frank feel calmer and more at peace with his decision, but it helped me and the others who were close to him cope better with losing him.

Letting Frank go was the hardest thing—I hope it's the hardest thing I ever do. But I never once questioned whether it was the right thing. Then or now.

Tom took a week and a half off after Frank's death, and when he got back "there was a patient who had been basically waiting for my permission to die. He didn't want to disappoint me after all my efforts to keep him going, and he needed to know I would be supportive of letting him go. That had a big effect on me." Now Tom makes sure to let his patients know what choices they have at the end of their lives.

I can just imagine how frightening it would be to be helpless and at everyone else's will and have no one as your advocate. Especially if you wanted to die. That would be worse than the physical pain. Here in San Francisco you can probably find someone to be on your side, but if you lived somewhere else— I think I'd leave home.

When it gets to the point that the ball game is over, I don't try to be rosy about it or present false hopes. As people get sicker, I check in with them, I ask them where they're at. I let them know when they're coming to a point where they're going to have to make choices. I tell them what I have that may help them, buy them more time, but I tell them what these treatments will or won't do to their quality of life. Those are the hardest discussions, but they're increasingly important as people with AIDS are living longer and at least a mild degree of dementia is often present in the later stages of the disease.

Sometimes Tom's honesty is appreciated. He told me about a mother who came to him after her son had died, and thanked him for telling her the truth "instead of saying, 'Here's this other thing we can throw at it.'" But occasionally his advocacy runs counter to a family's wishes for their loved one. Tom told me about a patient named Roger:

Roger had written to his mother to tell her that he was gay and had been diagnosed with ARC at that point. She had written back that she had torn up the letter, not shown it to the family, and he could consider himself disowned.

Six months later he had lymphoma, and then he went into a coma, and suddenly the mother showed up furious with what she called the horrible care he was being given, demanding we do everything to bring him back. I tried to explain that there was no sense to do any more than make him comfortable because any hope for recovery was gone and we could only prolong his agony. But I never got through to her. The rest of the family understood, but not her. It took Roger three weeks to die, and I believe it was because she wouldn't let him go. He was in and out of coma, and she was constantly there creating a scene.

If Tom had demonstrated annoyance at this demanding mother, or avoided her, or refused to engage with her, she would likely have become a bigger, not smaller problem, seeking alternative strategies to get her way. But Tom believed that if he went along with her in the face of what he knew was right for his patient, Roger would be the victim, and Tom as much a perpetrator as Roger's mother.

In such a case, it is often useful for the doctor to find another caregiver, someone skilled in family dynamics and psychosocial issues, to establish rapport with the challenging family member, and to act as a kind of liaison for the doctor, communicating information, helping the individual adapt to the reality of the situation. The liaison is not there *instead* of the doctor, but in addition to him or her. Often just the discussion of adopting such a plan of action will reduce tensions and enhance support for the patient. Of course there are no guarantees. Roger's mother's response to his dying was based on a lifetime's worth of emotion and experience with her son, and perhaps on important unresolved issues; she may have been immovable. But I performed such a role for years with cancer patients and their caregivers at the University of California Medical Center in San Francisco, and have seen its beneficial effects.

◂ ◂ ◂

Tom acknowledges that what motivates him to establish the kind of relationships that he does with his patients is more than altruism. He works in partnership with them; he is their advocate, to some degree because his work and his advocacy soothe his own wounds. Tom has needed support and solidarity from someone very important to him, and gotten judgment instead, and alienation.

My dad was raised in poor farming country in a corner of Appalachia by second-generation German parents with a strong work ethic. He had to quit school in the ninth grade to work on the farm, and his efforts were demanded, never rewarded. The concept of encouragement or praise didn't exist. This was the only way he knew, so he adopted the same approach raising his kids. He never once said he was proud of me or congratulated me. I was the first Eagle Scout from our little town and he had to be convinced to come to the awards ceremony. I was second in my high school class, and he wanted to know who was first.

I looked at getting into medical school as my last attempt to earn my dad's approval. When I got accepted to two medical schools and called home to tell him, he asked me if I knew what I was doing in choosing one over the other. I've recently been able to talk to him about these things, which has helped close the distance between us, even if the wounds haven't entirely healed.

Tom's 110 percent effort on behalf of his patients seems related to his yearning for approval from his father. It assures that they will not experience the kind of rejection he did. Tom's partnerships with his patients are his way of simultaneously supporting them and slowly healing the wounds that his father's remoteness may have caused.

✎ ✎ ✎

Many stories of caregiving relationships demonstrate for me that the biggest difference of all is the difference between zero and one, *zero* being the absence of a compassionate caregiver who is there for the patient as a partner in the healing process, and *one* being the presence of such a person. The absence contributes to the painful reduction of the patient to the status of an object or a problem. The presence of a caregiver does not necessarily elevate the patient, but compassionate care does affirm and honor the individual's humanity. Such care provides healing on other levels than the physical.

As this kind of caregiver, Tom relates to his patients as autonomous adults, not dependent children. He encourages their questions, he suggests alternatives to hospital routines that may ignore important needs of theirs. He is an especially strong advocate for his patients who are very ill, whose judgment and sense of identity may be impaired, or for whom attentive hospital care and clinical expertise may make the difference between life and death.

Hospitalization can be a terrifying experience for an individual. At the same time it can bond a patient and physician if the physician is responsive and caring. When someone close to the patient is angry or adversarial, such a bond may be vital to the patient. Tom told me a story that demonstrates the patient's need for advocacy, and how the physician may make a difference in such circumstances by breaking down barriers, or constructing protective buffers for the patient.

Geoff was like me in many ways, a doctor involved in AIDS health care. I felt immediately connected to him when we met in the middle of his illness. I met his parents during a prolonged hospitalization. His recovery was very slow with several complications. Geoff had been a trouper, but the course of medications was taking its toll. When I asked him if he felt depressed, his mother snapped, "He's not depressed, he's just feeling sorry for himself."

I only needed to see his face to know I had to get to work on his mother for everyone's sake. I told her that I'd be more worried if he wasn't somewhat depressed after what he'd been through, because that would simply be a denial of how ill he was. Her response was cold silence. I'm sure she knew I was addressing her denial more than Geoff's.

As his illness worsened, though, I witnessed a transformation in his mother. I had dreaded having to fend for both of us in discussing quality of life, and death and dying with his mother, but by then a great change had taken place. Her acknowledgment of his suffering, and her willingness not to prolong it—her intent listening to my suggestions of how to comfort him—were the one bright point in Geoff's demise.

A few months after Geoff's death, his parents asked to meet with me and I braced myself for the old mother. Instead I met a woman who expressed her emotions and her gratitude, and her recognition of the toll my work must take. When she left, she hugged me. The father, who had been very gentle and stoic all along, may have been the most grateful for the new wife he had, or maybe the one he had first married. They even came to my annual Christmas party where we make Christmas boxes of food and small gifts for AIDS patients.

Most of us are painfully aware that losses have the power to diminish us. But losses can also trigger transformation. Loss can liberate us from a too-narrow view of ourselves and what we do with our lives. Loss can nullify, at least for the moment, the restrictions we place on how we love and relate in the larger world. Relinquishing one's narrow view (of AIDS, of homosexuality, of the correct kind of doctor-patient or mother-son relationship) can be a wrenching experience. Somehow Geoff's mother must have let herself fully feel her grief at her son's dying. She must have, in a way, learned from her grief, to allow for a personal change of such significant dimension.

- - - -

I'm amazed at how often I have to tell a patient's family that he's gay, not to mention that he's dying of AIDS. When this happens, I try to keep the focus on the disease. Get them to think about the person's suffering. A lot of times families will try to put their anger and confusion aside. If they can't,

I try to explain that the person didn't tell them out of fear he would be rejected. I ask them please not to reject him now when he's dying. I tell them that's the ultimate fear, dying without them.

And I tell my patients what happens when you don't tell your family so that they have the chance to think about it beforehand. It may be painful to deal with now, but it's a whole lot more painful if you're dying or so sick that you can't deal with anything, and you have to handle your family's response to this kind of revelation on top of everything else. You don't want to do that. And you don't want to do that to me, either. I do play a little guilt trip there.

Tom's own family has accepted, if not embraced, the fact that he is gay. His mother came to see him to offer her support when Frank was dying—her first trip without Tom's father in fifty-one years of marriage. When Tom asked her and a sister he is particularly close to, to join him in Washington, D.C., in 1992 at the Names Quilt demonstration, his entire family showed up.

If someone asked me to picture my parents and sisters showing up for a candlelight march over that quilt, I couldn't fathom it. They don't understand my lifestyle all that well, but their acceptance has been pretty amazing. I think it was the best validation I could have that they loved me, that there were certain things that my being gay wouldn't interfere with.

✦ ✦ ✦ ✦

When I interviewed him, Tom was struggling with his own disability, a severe herniated disk that has required three surgeries and a long recuperation. He has had to close his practice temporarily, and it has been a challenge not to work. "For me, it's phenomenal," he told me.

Because it's so hard to give up work, Tom works on himself. Like many of the caregivers in these pages, he strives to understand how his own psychology influences his attitudes and actions as a caregiver, and his success with his patients. His convalescence is marked by introspection that cannot help but contribute to his healing and to his competence as a physician.

15

I Walked with Him to Death's Door

Gary Shepard is a caregiver who has chosen to devote himself to people in the last stages of AIDS. These are people who may be shutting down or opening up in ways they never have before. They are frequently engaged in what psychologists call "life review," which is looking back in an attempt to make sense of the twists and turns one's life has taken. They may be experiencing a profound sense of gratitude for love given and received in their lives; or they may be full of regret. Gary told me:

I just didn't know what to say the first time I sat with a person who was dying, and he said, "I'm sorry I lived my life the way I did. I really messed up parts of it. I wish I could do it over again—better, maybe." I've since discovered there's no answer to that kind of thing. The best thing you can do is just sit with that person.

It wasn't until I'd been doing the work about six years and had been with a lot of people who had died, that suddenly one day it hit me like a ton of bricks. I thought, what is the

189

purpose of my doing this if I can't hear what the message is? What are these people telling me?

Time after time, I'd sit with people at the end of their lives who were sorry that they had led their lives the way they did, or that they had held the values they had. Or I saw people blossom into wonderful spaces where they had not been before they were sick. And I thought a person shouldn't have to be dying to come to these realizations or find those wonderful spaces. My clients taught me that life isn't a rehearsal. That this is it. What we do *now*, how we act, what we believe, has consequences.

This work has changed me in a really profound way— Well, I don't know that it changed me. It unlocked me. I'm more authentic and more direct a person than I used to be. I have fewer secrets. I'm braver about being who I am.

Gary would not have used the word "brave" to describe himself some years ago. In the beginning of his caregiving experience as a Shanti volunteer, he was frightened.

I was working with a man named Howard and I only knew him five months, but it was a very intense five months. He had what I often refer to as diagnosis of the month. Every month it seems like he had something else—he had tubercular canker sores, he had KS lesions in his gums, he had CMV retinitis, you know—every month it was some big thing.

He was a person who relied on me pretty heavily because he had no support system. He was divorced with two children. His parents, his wife, they wouldn't be in the same room with him. They were afraid of catching the disease. So he was pretty much alone. And he relied on me a lot. I was on my knees holding his hands during a spinal tap one time. I changed his diaper. I did things you don't normally do for another adult.

I remember once sitting at home with my family eating dinner and the phone rang. It was Howard saying, "I'm bleeding from the rectum. Can you come and help me?"

I got up from the table, put on my coat, and as I'm driving over there I'm thinking, blood, infection, bleeding from the rectum. . . . But then I said, I can do this. Because if he's doing that, I can do this. I know it's going to be scary, and I know I can do it.

Gary demonstrates his commitment to his clients by his responsiveness. Their relationship is not merely an arranged marriage of the strong with the weak; it is a union of compassion, of prioritization. Gary doesn't even think about whether he will interrupt his dinner to help Howard in an emergency. He just goes. It's not that Gary's other responsibilities are irrelevant but that they lose their urgency in the face of Howard's suffering.

What is a so-called normal commitment for a caregiver in such circumstances? Each of us answers this question for ourselves, and the answer changes as a client's condition worsens due to illness, or as changes occur in the life of the caregiver. For Gary, the priority is the commitment; his primary considerations are how he will help, and how he will deal with his own fear.

〜〜〜

Dealing with fear, that of the person with AIDS and one's own, is often integral to the process of caregiving, as Gary learned for the first time with Howard.

At the end of Howard's life, the man who was taking care of him in the hospice called me and said, "I think it's a good day for you to come visit." I knew what that meant. I went over and they had him on a morphine drip and he was sort of comatose. A friend of his was there, the only other friend I ever knew that he had.

We both sat there, and I wasn't there very long before I realized how frightened I was. Howard had this sort of apnea where he would stop breathing, and then suddenly he'd start breathing again—this labored breath. And every time he stopped breathing, I got nauseous, got this awful feeling in my chest. I thought each time that he had died, and I was terrified of his dying. It went on for a couple of hours. He seemed stable in this kind of unstable way.

I finally went out to do some errands. When I came back, his friend left. So there I was in the room alone with him. And I realized that my job, my commitment to him, was to help him through the fearful parts. He had a lot of fear about dying alone. And it occurred to me that if I was afraid, he was afraid too; and that if I could find a way not to be afraid, maybe I could help him not be afraid. I think I did that by breathing, and by being open, and by reminding myself of my affection for him, and my agreements with him that I would be there for him.

I sat down next to the bed in a rocking chair that was there. Howard was lying on his side, facing me. And I just began to sing. It was purely intuitive. I began to sing songs I had sung to my kids when they were babies. In just two or three minutes his breathing changed dramatically, and I knew he was really dying.

I moved closer to him, sat on the edge of the bed and put my arms around him. I was as close as I could be to him, and I talked to him, into his ear. And suddenly he stopped breathing.

What seemed really profound to me was how we are people while we're alive, and we're not when we're gone. And that line between living and dying is so thin. I felt as if I had walked with him right up to the door, and he had to go through the door and I couldn't. And when he died, I stopped being afraid for him.

I felt he had given me this enormous gift—I've felt it since then with other clients, but this was the first time. Howard wasn't my brother, lover, husband or wife, and yet he had allowed me the privilege of being with him for his major life transition.

It made my own death seem less fearful. I thought, this is it. This is how it is. Someday I'll walk up to that door and someone else will see me through.

This was Gary's first client, the one he still thinks of nine years later. For many caregivers, the first client or patient, like one's first love, has a profound impact. Gary learned how to "be with" another person as a caregiver from Howard. In their five months together, he began to understand that it is possible to travel empathically into another person's experience, and to feel as if from the inside what life is like for him or her.

Gary didn't have to suffer all of Howard's fear of isolation and abandonment to understand it or to stand with Howard in the face of it. Gary could relate to abandonment from personal experience. His own father had died when Gary was thirteen, and in the wake of that, for all purposes, his mother had abandoned him and herself to grief. The depth of it frightened Gary: "My sense was that grief is this really disgusting thing that you avoid at any cost."

Gary wanted nothing more to do with death or grieving. After his father's funeral he decided he would never attend another, and he stuck to that decision for the next thirty years. He also refused to set foot inside a hospital, not even to visit friends or family.

On the surface, Gary seems like the last person to have committed himself to caring for people with life-threatening illnesses at all, let alone at the end of their lives; but below the surface, it makes perfect sense. Any one of us who has experienced abandonment, whether physical or emotional, through death, or divorce, or even unintentionally in the course of events, will crave safety, yearn for commitment, and dread further desertions. These are common human reactions and a common human fear known to some degree to just about all of us, and that degree intensifies as a result of abandonment.

In Gary's case, what his unconscious perceived as his parents' abandonment made him a particularly passionate caregiver. His unconscious remedy was to personify the opposite of abandonment. Providing safety and making the commitment never to desert the one he cares for is salve to his own wounds as much as to his clients'. When he tells Howard, "I'll never leave you, I'll be there till the end," Howard is soothed, and the remnant of the abandoned child who survives in Gary is comforted by the words as well.

～～～

It was a friend who introduced Gary to caregiving, someone who had just completed the Shanti training, and declared that it had changed his life and that he knew it would change Gary's too. "I think you should do it," the friend said. "You'd be incredible at it." But that wasn't why Gary was compelled to join Shanti Project.

> I think I was motivated by fear. At the time my oldest boy was around fifteen and my youngest about eight. I'd had sexual experiences with men outside my marriage, which my wife knew about, but I was otherwise in the closet. I couldn't talk to anyone about my fears. I was reading, almost surreptitiously, all this stuff in the papers about AIDS, and I was really scared that I had the virus and had given it to my wife, and we'd both die and leave my two kids abandoned.
>
> I remember making a conscious decision that I could run away from this fear, or I could run toward it, which seemed like the healthier thing to do. And I also thought that doing this training and then the work was like putting money in the bank. I just assumed there would be a time when I would need to call back the favor.
>
> But I had no idea what I was getting into. I spent the two training weekends crying, sometimes out of control.

The Shanti training is a profoundly moving experience. It is four and a half days of immersion into the world of people with AIDS, who describe the physical, emotional, and spiritual challenges they face and that their caregivers must face with them. At the time, believing that he might have AIDS, Gary was even more deeply affected by the case histories of the men and women he was meeting.

Trainees participate in an exercise called "In Memory Of," in which they are asked to bring a memento of a person they have lost, and to talk about that person to the group. Gary had brought something of his father's, whom he had not grieved in more than thirty years.

It was both strange and threatening to cry in front of other people. Gary had deplored the expression of grief, and had tried to avoid painful introspective explorations, and the Shanti training demanded exactly the opposite from him.

Now, as he continues to pursue a counseling degree, Gary sees how our denial works to protect us from experiencing the full extent of our grief or suffering, precisely because we are not equipped to deal with it all at once. As denial falls away and one's own pain is revealed in these tolerable increments, so does one's recognition of the suffering of the client in the caregiving relationship.

Gary believes that that recognition is crucial to his functioning as a caregiver.

> The first word that comes to my mind when I think of being with people who are in the dying process is the word "witness." I've always had this very strong feeling that as we suffer we need a witness—there has to be someone there who really sees how we suffer, and how much we suffer. For me it's like the tree falling in the forest. I think someone has to be there in order to hear the tree falling, and for my clients I am that person. I see it as part of my role.

Having performed this role many times for people in his care, Gary has gained the courage—a bit at a time—to bear witness to his own suffering. He recognizes its source as the death of his father, and his mother's emotional withdrawal from him, both perceived as abandonments by his thirteen-year-old psyche. In response, as Gary matured, it was important to him never to abandon anyone.

When he was eighteen, Gary began what would be a volatile, on-again, off-again, long-distance love affair with a girl from his hometown in Indiana. She never told him that she had gotten pregnant during one of his visits. It was three years after the fact that he learned she had had their baby and given it up for adoption.

> That was a horrible thing for me! That I wasn't there in the same way my father wasn't there for me. That was a predominant episode in my life, and I dreamed about it, and grieved over it for many years.

Gary had broken his vow that he would never abandon anyone. Never mind that he hadn't known about the child; the unconscious isn't impressed with excuses about what we know or don't know.

The episode hurt Gary, and it strengthened his resolve. Again he promised himself he would never abandon anyone; and one way he fulfills that promise is by making it his essential commitment to his clients. "I will never leave you," he says. "I'll be there with you at the end."

It took some time for Gary to trust in such fidelity. For him it takes a leap of faith to enter into any relationship because the possibility of abandonment is so painfully present. On the other hand, the need for relationship is especially sharp in one who has been abandoned.

Gary has regained a great deal of confidence in the human capacity to honor commitments and to stay present even during hard times. In his own life, he can point to a string of strong commitments: a twenty-five-year marriage, a twelve-year business partnership, nine years with Shanti Project.

✦✦✦✦

One of the most difficult aspects of caring for people with AIDS is how hard it is to anticipate the sufferer's physical circumstances from day to day, or even hour by hour. AIDS can wreak total havoc on strength and stamina in just that short amount of time. One tries to do the right thing: to honor the client's wishes; to engage with the client in "normal" activities; to eke out moments of pleasure in days of pain. But sometimes it's not so easy. Gary recalls:

> One of the worst days I've ever had as an AIDS caregiver was with a man named Mark. He wanted to do something nice for me, and he loved the grand gesture. He decided to take me out for lunch to a very nice restaurant.
>
> When I went to pick him up at his apartment I could see he wasn't well enough to be doing this. He had bad neuropathy and he walked with a cane, but not easily. At the restaurant he could hardly make it across the floor. We were quite a sight, me dragging this emaciated crippled man through this elegant restaurant. And he complained the whole time. The food wasn't right for him. He wasn't hungry.
>
> Back on his block in front of his building, I was trying to figure out how I was going to get him up the two flights of stairs, when he lost his balance and fell, skinning his hand, which started to bleed.
>
> Fortunately, Mark lived half a block from a hospital, and a physical therapist just happened to come upon us on her way to work. She knew exactly how to get a person up. I learned from her. She told me where to put my hands, where to put my weight, "Do this, do that"—and we had him on his feet.
>
> But I still had to get him up the stairs, and he could sense my fear. He was angry and agitated and humiliated. He rubbed his hand along the wall as we climbed, and smeared blood all the way up the stairwell. I had to go back down with a bucket and sponge and wash the blood off the wall.
>
> It was a terrible day and an out-of-control situation. I felt my own fear and personal inadequacy, which is a lot different from experiencing someone else's. And it shouldn't have hap-

pened. I should have said, "I'm sorry, we can't do this special lunch today because I don't think I can get you back up the stairs unless we have help." As it happened, Mark never went out again.

Gary's miscalculation in Mark's case is a result of his desire to help the one in his care live his or her remaining life to its fullest, for this is also part of the job for the devoted caregiver. Gary had deemed the potential rewards for Mark worth the risk of their outing, because of a similar excursion with Howard that had a happier ending.

One time I took Howard out of the hospital and down to the coast to a restaurant for dinner on a Sunday. He had to pull his oxygen machine with him into the restaurant. He had a patch on one eye from CMV, and he walked with a cane.

Common sense might have told me not to put us through it, but luckily common sense wasn't talking that day. For Howard, it was glorious. He was outside. He saw the ocean. He wasn't sick and dying; he was having dinner in a restaurant. He absolutely loved it. It was exactly the right thing to do.

In the last weeks and months of a person's life, doing the right thing may depend more and more on your intuition. But a cautionary note: some people with AIDS take the walk to death's door many times before passing through, and in between these visits may return to a relatively normal existence. It's important not to assume that the end is *here* when it's only near; it can be devastating for someone who is terribly ill and fighting desperately to survive to be treated as if he were dying.

It's vital to be attuned to your clients or patients, and as much as possible to let them indicate to you how they are and what they need. The tuning in to the patient-partner is another way of getting "inside" the other person's experience, and this approach opens doors inside ourselves. Another word of caution: these doors may open on our deepest fears.

Gary's deepest fear is of abandonment, and yet he has designed his life to confront abandonment over and over again, by volunteering to be with and care for people in their last weeks or months of life, people who are bound to leave him.

But at the same time, when Gary is there for each person as he said he would be, he affirms *from his own example* that abandonment is not the inevitable outcome of relationships. He begins to know that he can count on himself. And he increases his faith in a kind of karmic justice. Because he is constant in his commitment to be there for others, it is more and more likely that in his time of need, another will be there for him.

Ernest Hemingway wrote, in A *Farewell to Arms:* "The world breaks everyone and afterwards many are strong at the broken places," and he may as well have been writing about people like Gary, people who are willing to challenge their own deepest fears while helping another to do the same. Gary is becoming the very nurturing soul, the giving parent that his younger self had yearned for. In this way does the wounded healer heal himself, and at the same time provide his wounded partner with steadfast support.

— — —

You often hear people who do this work say that it's a pathway to spiritual life, or an opening to spiritual life. But I think sitting in a room with a progression of people with AIDS, and being a kind of container for their pain *is* the spiritual life. The pathway is how you got to that room.

For myself, I had to learn about grieving to get there. I didn't shed a tear when my own dad died. But now—I've learned how to cry.

I had a client named Bobby who had terrible dementia and it got to the point that he couldn't function any more. I had become friendly with his daytime attendant, and when it was time to move Bobby to a hospice, we were both there.

The ambulance arrived, and two men with uniforms

and gloves and masks walked in and picked up Bobby's little skinny body and put it into this chair. I had to go to the kitchen to cry. The images were just too overwhelming.

But Bobby's daytime caretaker was terrified that I was falling apart. I had to explain that this was how I *keep* from falling apart. I cry.

I've learned some other things: to strive for honesty in all things and with all people, to lay aside judgments— of myself and others. The reality is that people are different, and they deal with their pain differently, and you have to respect that.

I try to remain centered on the client, to empower the client, to love unconditionally. I ask myself, "What level of consciousness do I have to reach to understand this other person's reality?" It's a lesson I continue to learn, to forget, and learn again.

16
You Relapse a Lot

As a sophomore I was sixteenth in the nation among Catholic
schools as a one-meter spring board diver. I had this crew cut,
varsity letter sweater, cheerleader girlfriend, and all the time
I was shooting dope in the bathroom. I was an immediate
casualty of the drug culture. I smoked pot about six times and
then shot pharmaceutical cocaine. I had to spend six months
in an adolescent psych ward because they didn't have rehabs
for kids back then. I graduated high school from the Eastern
Pennsylvania Psychiatric Institute.

Richard Jackson knows a thing or two about self-destructive
behavior, having lived for long periods on the precipitous slope of
substance abuse, both of alcohol and IV drugs. But what was a lia-
bility has become an asset. His background makes him an especially
understanding caregiver for those people with AIDS who are part
of the street culture where drugs and alcohol are a way of life, and
for people who may have contracted AIDS by needle sharing—as
Richard believes he did—because he knows that people like

himself can take a slide into darkness, and rebound to a higher quality of life than they knew before. That's how it has been for him.

◢ ◢ ◢

Richard grew up in Atlantic City, New Jersey, formerly a summer resort, now a tough gambling town where "dog eat dog" has always been the ruling ethic, and "people were victims or they were victimizers." Richard never knew his father. His mother left him and his brother with her parents when she remarried, and his grandparents adopted Richard when he was six years old. Although it couldn't compensate for the experience of being abandoned by both his birth parents, life with his grandparents was one of comparative privilege: his grandfather served twelve years as city commissioner, and then as mayor of Atlantic City for two terms in the 1960s.

Meanwhile, Richard attended high school leading the double life of an all-American teenage addict, managing to pull himself together when he had to. In this way, in spite of his stint in the psychiatric hospital, he applied and was accepted to the University of South Carolina. And there he discovered karate.

> I grabbed karate like a drowning person grabs a life raft. I got through college and competed in tournaments, and I was good. I got involved in professional karate after that, and then full contact karate—kick boxing. I was forced to retire as the number one contender in the world in the featherweight division because the drug addiction took over again.
>
> I ended up back in New Jersey and went to work for the casinos. There were nine casinos and I got fired from seven of them because my work at each of them interfered with my other work, which was my full-time job maintaining my addiction. Way more important a job! Takes way more hours! Everything else got in the way. I went from dealing blackjack and craps at the best casino in Atlantic City to the bottom of the barrel.

I spent days in houses with no doors, no windows, no electricity, shooting up over and over again, sharing needles. I knew I was probably HIV positive and there were other people the same way. But the drugs are the most important. I couldn't find my way out. That's what addiction is about.

It was from the bottom of the barrel that Richard began the long, slow climb back to a better life. "Bottoming out" is a common experience in the cycle of addiction. It occurs when life is no longer manageable, when basic survival needs aren't being met. The feeling of powerlessness is overwhelming, and blatant self-destructive behavior may commence, like Richard's stint in Atlantic City shooting galleries. The addict experiences a true dark night of the soul.

For some people, hitting the bottom breaks their fall. From this place it is possible to rebound, as Richard did. (Some people in the recovery movement believe it's *necessary* to touch bottom to recover.) But others may not recover from their fall, and some may not want to even *try* recovery. Richard remembers one of his first assignments as an AIDS counselor on San Francisco General Hospital's Ward 5A, a man who made him question what he knew and didn't know about recovery.

Brian was twenty-one, lived on the streets his whole life. He's real sick, and he's telling me about his chronic speed use, and injecting speed and anything else he can get his hands on.

Of course, I tell him he needs to not use and things will get better, because that's what I know. And he says to me, "I have zero T-cells. I've had a million infections. I'm sick as a dog. I have to prostitute myself to live. I'm waiting for the next person on the street to sneeze in my face and kill me. Why do I want to get sober?"

I was floored by that. I realized that what I'd said to him was ridiculous. Things probably aren't going to get better for Brian. And whatever it takes to enable him to get a job, get an apartment, be responsible, and do all those things we call "sobriety" in the recovery community—I don't think he's got time for all that.

By his fifth hospitalization, I'd learned to just be there with him. I didn't suggest going to meetings. I didn't suggest trying not to use today. All I did was try to listen to him and key in on the positive things he talked about. Something positive that he had done for himself or for somebody else, or that somebody else had done for him. It was a wonderful lesson for me.

The lesson taught Richard several things about AIDS caregiving: the value of just being there; that you can't "fix it" for your client; that as dark and difficult as a life may be, it still may be shot through with positive moments, and that sometimes acknowledging and reinforcing these may be enough. And he learned that "recovery," as he has known it, doesn't happen for everyone.

✦ ✦ ✦

I went into recovery because I was tired of losing stuff— like relationships—which tells you I had them to lose. At a certain point I decided I didn't want to lose whatever stuff I had left.

Now I deal with people who don't have any stuff to lose. AIDS patients who are disenfranchised, third-generation homeless, have nothing. Telling them to wait till they bottom out before they go into recovery is useless. They're not going to bottom out. The bottom is the bottom. It's not going to get any worse. They're going to be dead.

It's confronting the exact opposite of what worked for me. That's been a challenge for me. It's difficult for me to talk to patients who are actively using. Someone tells me he's got a gram of speed at home waiting for him as soon as he gets out of the hospital. I want to say, "Let me go home with you and we'll throw that out. You need to be clean and sober." But I don't say it.

Having been through a lot of rehabs myself, and dealing with counselors and psychiatrists and psychologists who weren't alcoholics, I remember carrying a banner like, "You don't know what I'm going through." And it's true, they didn't. Now I try very hard to keep an open mind and not to judge.

Richard's recovery began in 1985. "It was a turbulent period, trying to get sober and stay sober. I was doing twelve-step meetings, couple's counseling, and then I got my HIV diagnosis." In 1985, a diagnosis of HIV was the equivalent of an AIDS diagnosis, and an AIDS diagnosis "was the equivalent of a death notice."

Early on, trying to get sober is kind of like being a round ball trying to fit into anything other than a round space. Your nerves are firing and nothing feels right. You relapse a lot.

I couldn't talk about my HIV status in Narcotics Anonymous (NA) meetings or AA meetings—at Alcoholics Anonymous (AA) they were talking about doing away with holding hands at the prayer at the end because of AIDS. I'm supposed to go in, raise my hand and say, "Hey, I'm Richard, I'm an alcoholic, and I had a good day today—I didn't drink." But I wanted to say, "Bullshit. I had a fucking horrible day. I have AIDS!" But there was nobody to tell.

The woman Richard lived with during his early attempts at recovery tested negative for HIV. He credits this relationship with "keeping me alive" in those days. She helped him find an HIV-support group.

The group was nearly 100 percent gay men, so I was always kind of on the fringe. All the guys did was talk about what some other guy was wearing, or how somebody looked, or who was sleeping together. They were just trying to figure out how to live normal lives with this disease. Relationship and sex were big issues for me, too, but mainly I kept going back because it was the only place where I could talk about

HIV. I didn't know any recovering junkies that were HIV positive or had AIDS. The only people I knew with AIDS were gay, middle-class, white men. Outside of the hour and a half I spent at the group each week, I never saw them.

✐ ✐ ✐

One thing Richard learned from his HIV-support group, and all his other groups, was that he wanted to talk about his HIV status. Eventually it was his unwillingness to lie about it anymore that signaled a real change in direction for Richard, and in 1992 brought him to San Francisco.

I wanted to be able to interview for a job and be honest about my HIV status. I knew that if I couldn't do it in San Francisco, then there was no place on this earth I could. I wanted to be around those other zebras.

So I ended up out here. I applied to twenty different places, and the first one I interviewed for I lied through my teeth about my status! I got the job—in drug and alcohol rehabilitation—and quit the same day. I just wasn't interested in doing any more recovery work.

Fortunately, one of the twenty applications Richard filled out was for Shanti Project as an AIDS counselor on San Francisco General's Ward 5A. At first, in spite of all he knew about HIV disease, Richard wasn't prepared for what he saw—for the severe, debilitating symptoms that can accompany advanced AIDS. But the Shanti model said that Richard could help just by listening. He didn't have to do anything except be nonjudgmental and share what he knew from his own experience in counseling and recovery.

The challenge was, could I do that? I didn't have any crutches. I didn't have any painkillers. I had to be out there without my old coping skills that had been taken away.

All the things that other caregivers do, I had to do. I had to go to a caregivers' support group. I had to talk, talk, talk about the things that scared me on the ward, about the horrible sights—people with monstrous-looking KS, people bleeding, people not being able to breathe. I had to talk about it rather than not talk about it. Where I'd come from, you shoot a bag of dope, get drunk, don't deal with anything difficult.

Now the situation is totally reversed. Now it's deal with that person's KS because you need to; deal with it and be healthy with it.

Richard says he feels just a step or two ahead of the people he cares for, people who don't believe they'll ever be loved or cared for or make any positive contribution or difference in the world. They may well concentrate on the pain they can control rather than the pain they can't control. In this way they demonstrate some power, even if it is just over the terms of their own unhappiness. Understanding firsthand their disappointment, their manipulative behavior, their mistrust of health professionals and the health care system, Richard was primed to meet the challenges they presented. He was also sensitive to the fact that some IV drug users are uncomfortable with the religious orientation of some recovery programs, or support groups that consist mostly of women, or mostly of gays, or straights, or whatever group contributes to the user's feeling of separation or difference.

Moralizing about the evils of substance abuse, admonishing one to grab hold of his bootstraps, may be just the wrong thing to say to someone trapped in addictive behavior. Well-intentioned social service agencies often ignore the intelligence, experience, and creativity of their clients, all of which are resources for restoring the equilibrium we call health. Searching for psychological insights into addiction or treating it as a symptom of some form of psychopathology may be so much wheel spinning to the user, for whom such considerations are far less important than their next drink or fix, or where they're going to sleep tonight, or whether they will eat today, or the progress of their disease.

◢ ◢ ◢

Everyone has a different story—Richard speculates that an absent father and a mother who left him and a genetic predisposition to alcohol contributed to his. But everyone's story is also the same. Whatever the source of the original wound, the user seeks pain relief in alcohol or drugs. Of course, their use only increases their sense of powerlessness and separation.

These two fears, of abandonment and powerlessness, are common emotions among IV drug users. Sometimes they are terribly difficult for the human psyche to bear, in which case they are rarely experienced directly. Anger is often a defense against these fears, turned inward if we believe we are responsible for our painful situation, or outward, onto parents, or society, or institutions, depending on where we place the blame. Unsuspecting caregivers may find themselves the brunt of a client's anger, or subjects of their client's manipulation. Clients who feel hopeless, who resist trusting in their caregivers, or who believe that manipulation is the only way to get their needs met can severely tax caregiver resources. You have to learn how to let such clients be angry with you, or disappointed in you, without feeling guilty or taking the anger or disappointment personally.

For people who are homeless and desperate, abandoned or rejected by family and society, without the strength or support to pull themselves back up, embarrassment and humiliation may be the companion of their other miseries. No matter how the user handles his or her pain, no matter whether anger or self-obsession or humiliation and despair accompanies it, caregivers can move the client who is immobilized by insecurity and self-recrimination by caring openly about him or her, by not participating in finding fault or placing blame, by acknowledging the problems, by focusing on the positive, and in that way helping to create a context for hope.

Hope connects us to an attitude of optimism toward life that is absolutely necessary in order to balance despair or even face one's pain. And facing one's pain is the key to healing. Unfortunately, for many streetwise people who have become junkies and alcoholics and are HIV positive, their experience tells them not to set themselves up for more disappointment. They dare not hope. They deny instead.

Even the most resilient of us deny parts of our reality that we find painful and don't want to deal with. Denial may give us time to regroup psychologically after catastrophic news. Denial is necessary for survival, a way to ward off desolation or panic. Caregivers have to understand their client's need to look away from certain realities. But when denial becomes an active agent of destruction, by chronically concealing the high costs of one's self-destructive behavior or the reality of one's HIV disease, then it does become a problem. People employing denial in this way, as Richard did, may resist assistance for many years. Eventually, after telling and retelling one's painful stories as a way of gradually suspending denial, the individual may finally make the connection between his use of narcotics or alcohol and the negative situations in his life, and then he can begin to break the cycle of self-sabotage—though the process may be bitter enough to challenge even the most skilled caregivers.

✐ ✐ ✐

Richard's clients can face their pain only in proportion to their hope. When they believe Richard's promise to help, they may let go a little. More often, however, they continue to resist help because of their strong sense that caring comes with a price tag. Inevitably, they will be disappointed by their caregivers who can't fix it for them, who don't have all the answers, and who aren't able to protect them from the assaults of HIV disease.

Sympathetic caregivers with the best intentions may try to protect the client from confronting the destructive consequences of his or her drug or alcohol use, or the painful feelings associated with such consequences. In such cases, though they are clearly enthusiastic supporters of their clients, their efforts on behalf of the user will fail for sure, in spite of the most caring intentions and enthusiasm, if there isn't a treatment program or process geared to change the destructive behavior. And eventually, when the client's use of drugs continues, the caregiver is likely to become angry and frustrated, or feel victimized by the client's behavior. Then everybody loses. Caregivers should be prepared for how challenging and intractable addiction can be—perhaps even more so when combined with HIV disease.

It is equally true that the best, most proven treatment program or process will also fail if it lacks genuine caring, support, and enthusiasm.

Significant progress, like Richard's, occurs when both a process and support exist, *and* the client is highly motivated to suspend his denial and acknowledge his problem, and is sincerely committed to the agreed-on program. In the absence of all these ingredients, the volunteer caregiver or health professional can still listen, and provide an ongoing supportive presence.

> I come from a background where the process wasn't important, the results were important. It meant more to my grandfather that my brother and I get A's in school—with him doing our homework—than for us to do our own homework and get C's.
>
> Now I've learned that the process is what's important. Life for me is a process now; it's not about achieving some end. It's the best job in the world for me right now. And it's a real change for me, to be able to listen to somebody tell me something that I know from my own experience is wrong, and to sit there and listen and acknowledge the person who's talking to me, and respect him for the process he's going through. I think it's one of the most important things that's happened to me in this work.

One of the programs that Richard subscribes to is "harm reduc-tion," a relatively new model of addiction treatment in the United States. He uses an analogy to describe it:

> When you have a damaged freeway overpass, cracked, but still standing, you don't rush in and tear it down. You either shore up the existing overpass, or build a temporary overpass alongside the damaged one and then repair, or remove and rebuild the original.
>
> Most traditional models of alcohol and drug treatment are moral models. They shame you into acting the right way. They take away your prop and build you up from there. From an engineering standpoint, it's not necessarily the best treatment.

Harm reduction recognizes that there may be stages to achiev-ing abstinence. Methadone maintenance is an example of harm reduction. The crutch is not kicked out from under. The process focuses on reducing harm gradually.

> You educate users about cleaning their works, about sharing needles. If your client pays for his or her drugs by prostituting, suggest they get their first trick of the night to pay for a hotel room. That way they have a safe place to take the rest of their customers. You take little steps like that, and then at some point you make a contract with your client: "We meet once a week. Could you not come high to our meeting?" And so on.

＊＊＊

As talented as Richard is in caring for the special needs of the substance user, he was surprised to discover his facility for affecting his clients' families. He was surprised because he had been alienated for long periods from his own family—except for his older brother.

I could always find out some tidbit of information about what was going on in the family through him. He was there for me for my entire time of using, although he didn't approve of it. He was a policeman in Atlantic City. I'd bang on his window in the middle of the night and he'd say, "I can't believe you're doing this," and take a gold chain off from around his neck so that I could sell it to get a fix. There are people who would call that "enabling." I call it helping. That's how he knew to make the pain go away for me. I love my brother for that.

When many years later, Richard met the sister of a drug addict who had just died on Ward 5A, he was, perhaps, especially attentive when she poured out her heart to him.

Skip had been estranged from his family for years and years, except for this one sister he had always maintained some connection with. She told me how much she loved her brother and how much he had hurt everybody in the family by how he lived and what he became. In light of my personal experience, it was an incredible thing to stay open to.

Now the family was all gathering, and there was a lot of disagreement about who was going to be in charge, who would make the arrangements, who would do this, who would do that. The sister was furious that after all these years the family was taking over, when she didn't believe they really cared.

I told her I understood how angry and hurt she must feel that no one acknowledged what she had done—holding the family together, being the thread that connected them with her brother, who was still part of the family, whatever he'd done. And then I suggested that if her brother's death caused her family to experience a minute or a second of true caring for him, then maybe that was good. I knew she didn't think they deserved to be part of his death, and I was asking her to let them be. I knew I was taking a chance. When Skip died most of the family was there around his bed, holding hands.

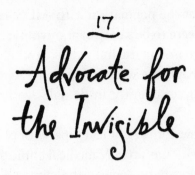

17

Advocate for the Invisible

Any agency or individual can call on me to help any woman or child in Marin County who is HIV positive. People assume that if you live here you've got all sorts of money, yet we have a very large homeless population. Part of my daily struggle is to figure out how to get this individual or that one off the streets and into some kind of housing. We also deliver hot meals and groceries to people. I have clients who have nothing.

Marin County, less than an hour's drive north of San Francisco, is one of the wealthiest communities in the United States, renowned for hot tubs, redwood forests, New Age philosophy, and upward mobility. Few people know that this county of approximately 250,000 has the second largest AIDS population per capita in California. San Francisco is first, Los Angeles third.

Marin boasts a score of charming little towns typical of others throughout America, where the population feels safe and removed from the possibility of AIDS, when, in fact, it exists next door and downtown. AIDS is an equal opportunity virus. Its seeming invisibility has to do with a community's denial, and it is, unfortunately,

quite common. For the population with AIDS in such communities, there might seem to be safety in anonymity; but anonymity or
invisibility tends to isolate the individual. And it may be more of a
risk than many people are willing to take to "come out" as being
HIV positive in a community in denial, even to access much-
needed services.

Penny Chernow, former clinical supervisor of the Marin AIDS
Project's Specialty Clinic, an HIV medical clinic at Marin General
Hospital, is an advocate for some of these invisible people, in particular, women with AIDS in Marin County. Penny arranges to
have a baby taken care of while mom sees the doctor, or she
arranges for the doctor. She finds rides, or day care for mothers with
AIDS, or establishes a support group for HIV-positive women, or
helps a woman tell her teenage son about her diagnosis.

> Everyone else in her life knew, but she was too frightened
> to talk to him about it. It took three months of weekly group
> meetings with other mothers sharing how they told their
> children and close family, and her practicing with us how
> to tell him.
>
> The fear is that the child won't be able to deal with the
> news. It's a pretty tough message: "I'm here to take care of
> you, but I'm going to leave you before you're done needing
> my care." For young children especially, that's about as fright-
> ening as it gets. The parent wants to soothe the child and
> say, "I'm okay, I'm healthy, I'm not dying right now." But she
> doesn't want to lie to the child, either. There's also the fear
> that the child will reject you because you're leaving, or that
> the child will become terribly depressed or unmanageable
> around this news.
>
> Fortunately, because of the preparation, I think, this
> mother's conversation with her son went well.

∕ ∕ ∕ ∕

In the early 1980s, Penny was married, her five children were
grown, and she was looking for something to do:

I didn't want to work full time, but I wanted something that would challenge me emotionally and mentally. I had worked with abused women before. I had a degree in psychology, so I had some experience in social service.

I thought about volunteering to do AIDS-related work, but I wasn't really sure I could do it. I was afraid I'd get too connected. I was not looking to invite grief into my life if I could avoid it. What pushed me over the edge was reading Randy Shilts's *And the Band Played On* when it first came out. I was outraged by what he wrote about—the homophobia, our government's lack of caring, the blood bank scandal, about some people's reactions—talking about concentration camps, talking about it being God's punishment. I had to get involved.

Penny went back to school and earned a master's degree in women's psychology and began to see the need for women's advocacy among people with AIDS. When her volunteer work at Marin AIDS Project grew to forty-plus hours a week it became a full-time job, and then a paid position.

The urge to be involved in some good work, to make a difference, is a motivating force for many people who get into AIDS work. But "making a difference" begins to pale as a motivation after too many days spent with babies with AIDS, or with dying mothers who want, and don't want, to transfer the care of their babies to someone else. Then, to stick it out, you have to find a healthy way of identifying with your client. Penny's history provided painful moments enough for her to appreciate her clients' suffering and society's negligence toward them.

I grew up in an intact family, but with major neglect. My father was a physician and my mother was a nurse and they were both very busy and not much interested in any of their children, even when we were small. I remember feeling hungry often, and wearing unlaundered clothes in early elementary school. No one expected this sort of thing from a

physician and his wife. I actually grew up poor. My parents
had money but they never shared it, so I understand something about poverty. And because they rarely paid attention
to me, I grew up feeling invisible—and I repeated that pattern
in marrying a man who also wasn't real interested in who I
was—so invisibility is an important part of my history, and
maybe why I identify so much with my "invisible" clients.

After two years working with the Marin AIDS Project, Penny's
husband of twenty years left her. "He couldn't deal with the fact
that I was working with people who were dying. We were both
middle-aged, but for him the subject was a little too real," she told
me. "That was a major wound for me."

I understand from that what it feels like to get news that
changes your whole world, what it feels like when reality
as you knew it disappears. I understand grief. I understand
depression. I took to my couch for six months. I liked
dark rooms.
    I learned something about caregiving from it, though.
I learned I didn't want to be around those people who said,
"What's the matter with you? Get up! You can do this, you
can do that!" I couldn't wait to get those people out of my
house and out of my face. I told them, "Look, I can't do
anything right now. I'll call you when I'm better."
    I was completely torn apart. I wasn't sure I was going
to survive it. The people who helped me most were those
who trusted that I would. I had one friend who came over
after work two or three nights a week and sat in the dark
with me and held my hand. He never said, "Did you eat
something today?" He never said, "Why don't you do something, volunteer, read a book?" He just sat with me and
held my hand. I loved having him there. I didn't want to
talk, I didn't want to entertain him, and I didn't want him
to entertain me, but I needed the physical connection.

Penny applied this knowledge to her caregiving. Now when she enters a darkened room, she doesn't rush to open the blinds to let the sunshine in. When you're in turmoil inside, when you're jolted by shock or grief, it can feel soothing to cut down on stimulae from outside your mind, even sunlight. Penny doesn't bustle around. "You come in quietly. You feel the situation." She respects another's silence. She says to someone who is noncommunicative, "I'm here and I'm just going to sit with you. I'm going to trust that if there's something I can do for you, you'll let me know."

Caregiving has been a learning process from the beginning, an ongoing education, and a humbling one:

> I always thought I knew so much about what people needed. For instance, I used to get very upset when a client refused to go on AZT, which isn't for everyone, of course, but I thought it was at the time.
>
> Now I understand that you've got to be where the client is: If the client believes she's going to "be here for the cure," or that brown rice is the answer, you've got to support that. Not by encouraging it, not by saying, "Eat more rice," or "Of course you're going to be here for the cure," but by not challenging her beliefs.
>
> They need to believe. My experience is that when and if a person stops believing in whatever, or if or when they get sick enough and tired enough, then they'll cross over to dying. I believe the disease itself crosses them over. You won't have to. And you have to trust that they'll get there in plenty of time to take care of things. And if they don't, so what? They've got to die the way they want to. It's their last piece of dignity, their last choice.
>
> But if you walk in with an agenda of what they ought to believe, or what they ought to know, or how much denial is healthy, you're going to burn out quicker than they will.

So if Penny's client is feeling great and thinks she's going to live forever, they talk about her plans and her good feelings. The next day if she comes in saying, "I've got fevers. I really don't think I'm going to make it through the month," Penny asks if there are any important things that need attention, any things the client wants to finish up? And a week later when the woman comes in feeling great again, it's cause for celebration. "I don't need them to be consistent," Penny says. "They need me to be consistent. My role is support and advocacy for whatever they need, which changes because their health changes. I need to be able to go with that."

> I've also learned how important it is to tell people positive things. I always verbalize my warm feelings toward someone, or my positive responses. I don't assume they know that I think they're terrific. I know as a neglected child—and even now—I can't hear that kind of positive reinforcement enough. I need to know that you see what's good about me.

Penny has relied on her experience to guide her caregiving. When she began to move from one-on-one volunteer work to group work, it was new territory. Penny found out, as so many other caregivers have, that you learn by doing.

> Three years ago, I started a women's support group in Marin. At that time we had about ten women on our caseload at the Project. One of them was a young, vital woman who was very eager to meet other women with HIV. She didn't know any, and felt very isolated. She came to my group every week for a year, and was the only one who showed up.
>
> After a year I finally got it. I called all the women I knew who were HIV positive and said, "I've got this woman, she comes every week, she feels so isolated, she'd really like to meet someone who is HIV positive. Would you mind coming next week just to talk to her?" And they all showed up. They couldn't wait to be there for her! What I learned from this is that women are raised to be nurturers for everybody but themselves.

The group has now taken on a life of its own. The women share everything: hopes, fears, literature, information. When one goes on a new experimental drug, they're all intensely interested. They're also very interested in nutrition and health.

Penny's point that women tend to nurture everybody but themselves is crucial to successful caregiving for women with AIDS. A woman who has three little children to round up and dress and take with her on the bus because she can't afford a sitter and doesn't have a car, is likely to skip her doctor's appointment. Managing her own health care will come second to managing her children, which is often viewed as "noncompliance" by medical caregivers.

If her primary medical provider is a public clinic, a woman may have to wait as much as two or three hours to see a doctor; and since very few public clinics do gynecological exams, she may have to wait another two or three hours at another location for those. If she has children with her, she's not likely to wait—unless she has backup support that she can count on, someone she trusts who can look after her kids while she's out.

These women are frequently their children's sole support. They are women who are making decisions vital to themselves and their children without a whole lot of information or input or experience, and they are doing it alone. Caregiving agencies are only beginning to reach out to these women, and are discovering that they are ill-equipped to serve them.

━ ━ ━

For the past decade and a half of the AIDS pandemic, our caregiving models have been male oriented, and women's unique needs have not been adequately addressed. Penny thinks the emphasis on emotional support over practical support in many caregiving training programs is one of the symptoms of this.

The way to reach our women tends to be through their

children, rather than becoming friends like we've done with men. Our "buddy system," if you will, has been based on matching a volunteer and a client. They start out with phone calls before they meet face to face, and they get to know each other over time.

For women, what works better is when you can come in and do something constructive for them—babysit for them, give them respite from child care.

As I said, women have a hard time accepting nurturance for themselves. We have to find other ways of connecting with them, and practical support is one way.

In Western societies, mastery and nurturance have been generally seen as in opposition. Men have been charged with mastery, women with nurturance.

Historically, women's de-emphasis of mastery as motivation may have to do with the fact that the dominant male society that reveres mastery does not value women, and often devalues their nurturance and caregiving. Women, and many men, are offended by this dominant male model because they find little love in it. In such societies, people seem to have forgotten the higher purpose of community—to support (nurture) its membership—in favor of proving which among its members are the most powerful or the most accomplished.

I find Penny's observations very interesting as they relate to the old mastery versus nurturance debate. In caregiving, emotional support is sometimes distinguished from practical support, and caregivers may choose to provide one or the other, although there's plenty of overlap. Still, emotional support is considered the charge of the peer counselor who is there to listen, to understand, to hold the hand of the client in distress, while practical support generally consists of help with chores like grocery shopping, or laundry, or scrubbing the bathroom floor.

Emotional support may be seen as a refined form of nurturance. You'd think women would identify with it most. But in fact, many women prefer more practical support, perhaps because it brings them closer to mastering their situation. Here, mastery is not the opposite of nurturance, but its complement. Clearly, it's time to develop new models of AIDS caregiving based on the real needs of men and women.

Advocates and caregivers like Penny have integrated their own capacities for mastery and nurturance in their efforts to improve the lives of people with AIDS. In Penny's case, her work has provided her a tremendous boost to her sense of self. She has a sense of what she can accomplish, of what is possible. In fact, she is becoming a master at the work. And this feeds an ongoing healing process, not only for those people who come under her care, but also for herself as she continues to make outstanding caregiving her definition of success.

✦ ✦ ✦

Among the mothers in Penny's groups, their children, whether HIV positive or negative, are most often their top priority. Their own treatment for AIDS is a secondary concern. For women without children, a love relationship is often the top priority. When any of the women in Penny's groups established a new relationship, all of the women experienced a burst of hope for themselves. In general, the concerns of these women reflect the context of their lives. Depending on their circumstances, conversation at a women's support group may range from the latest herbal remedy, to violence at home.

Interestingly, heterosexual men with AIDS are as concerned for their love lives, and as fearful about an absence of love in their futures as women and gay men with AIDS. They want to know, "How will I tell someone I meet that I'm HIV positive and not have her run away screaming?"

There's a lot of invisibility that heterosexuals with AIDS have to contend with. There just aren't that many programs for them, social events, even safe sex videos. Try to find a safe sex video for a heterosexual that doesn't look like the Surgeon General's report! But there's got to be a hundred of them for gay men that are absolutely great. It makes safe sex look so exciting you can't wait to go out and try it!

Too often, in addition to heterosexuals with AIDS, another victim of society's blind eye is the child of a person with AIDS. Penny remembers a mother with AIDS whose husband had died of the disease two years earlier, but whose child was HIV negative.

While the mother was working, the child went to day care, but now she's gotten sick and can't work, and so can't pay for day care. Now, we could move this little guy out of this place he's been for two years, where he knows everybody and feels safe, and put him into a free program; or we could figure out a way to finance the day care he's in now and not change his life any more than we have to at the moment.

But because the boy is HIV negative, I couldn't get any funding! If he had been positive, I'd have had it in a minute! I called every agency you can name, and finally got funding for three months through Season of Sharing [the *San Francisco Chronicle*'s Christmas fund-raiser for needy people]. When those three months are up, I'll be back on the trail.

It's a perverse kind of reverse discrimination. Penny's HIV-positive children go right to the head of many people's lists, day care included. She knows several organizations that have set aside funds for these children, but they are not for kids who are HIV negative with a positive parent.

✔ ✔ ✔

Caring for HIV-positive kids, or for kids whose parent is HIV positive, is often a special challenge. Money, for their medication if they're sick, or for day care or sitters if their parent is sick, is only part of it. The mother with an HIV-positive five-year-old who requires medication, isn't going to find her babysitter on the local high school bulletin board; she needs a trained caregiver.

AIDS orphans are an even bigger challenge to the community:

> Most foster care parents won't take kids with AIDS, especially babies. There's still a major fear of casual contamination, and when you consider that babies have no control over bowels or bladder, and that even in 1995 people aren't sure what "bodily fluids" we're talking about when we talk about risk factors—for instance, even though we know that urine doesn't carry appreciable amounts of the HIV virus, people are scared of changing diapers.

In coming years, as AIDS continues to affect the heterosexual community, we will see increasing numbers of AIDS orphans. Today worldwide, there are more children orphaned by AIDS than there are people living with AIDS. World Health Organization projections are that the number of AIDS orphans will reach 10 million in five years. In the United States, projections are that 72,000 to 125,000 children under age eighteen will fall into that category by the year 2000, and 30,000 of them will live in New York City.[1] Agencies and individuals are beginning to address this problem with suggestions for "permanency planning" that encourages parents with AIDS to acknowledge their situation to themselves and to their families, and to begin to plan for their children's welfare after their death. Questions such as "What will become of the children?" may be impossible to answer, but "Where will they go, who will care for them, and what kind of support can they expect from the State?" are all important to ask. And although some of the answers may be as tough as the questions, there are some answers to be found.

These are the kinds of questions that Penny has devoted herself to finding answers for.

> I'm good at looking at things and saying, "Okay, what's possible here?" For example, every caregiving agency has a durable

power of health or durable power of attorney that people fill out that designates a caring person whom they trust to step in and direct what will happen to them when they're not able to do so. This takes some of the burden off the sick person, and gives them the security of knowing they'll be taken care of in the way they want.

Yet no such document exists for mothers to designate what will happen to their children when they're too sick to care for them any more.

Penny sees "durable power" as it exists now as another expression of caregiving conforming to a male model. "My challenge is to bring us up to speed for women's needs," she says. She is at work on a prototype document designed for the parent with AIDS for distribution among AIDS agencies.

The numbers alone ensure that the special needs of women and children in the world of AIDS will not remain invisible for long, and Penny predicts that the children affected by HIV will change our volunteer forces. But she hates to wait for the natural flow of events to nudge us toward realization and action.

Right now volunteers aren't screened for histories of sexual abuse. This has got to be changed. And screening for TB is only now just beginning.

I see our volunteer teams training a special force for women and children. I'd like to see more active recruitment around that.

✦ ✦ ✦ ✦

Caregiving is an evolving set of aptitudes, and in this first decade and a half of caring for people with AIDS, we can chart some of the changes that have occurred. One of the primary changes has been in the life expectancy of people with the disease. Previously, caregivers could count on serving people who were dying of AIDS, which meant going through the psychological and emotional processes associated with dying: anticipatory grief, let-ting go, settling unfinished business as a means of seeking closure and lending coherence to the life already lived.

Now caregivers are more likely to be caring for people who are living with the disease. A bout with PCP or Kaposi's sarcoma used to be fatal. Now both can frequently be managed with medical intervention. These days, more and more, caring for people who are living with AIDS means supporting men and women with a sur-vivor's mentality who have taken the position that they might make it, or they might not, but they won't stop trying. Such clients are inspirations to their caregivers.

Anyone who has been living with AIDS is a survivor, and cer-tainly those who are living symptom-free with HIV or an AIDS diagnosis and whose quality of life has not been compromised are too. Survivors are those who have contracted any of the seemingly endless infections that are associated with AIDS, and rebounded; and they are also those who are determined to make it through the day, day after day, and do.

For some, the ordeal of survival has become an experience of healing and growth. I have seen many people surviving with AIDS who speak poignantly of a sense of possibility and self-efficacy learned through their years of living with the disease. The fact that one has survived a bout with pneumocystis, may mean that she or he has learned to cope more effectively with the curse of helpless-ness and come out the other side, back to a greater sense of control. That such a change is possible is something not every caregiver knows, and the knowledge that one can at times come back, from even the darkest places, is enlightening.

I don't mean that psychological factors carry more weight in the healing process than physical realities, such as methods of medical treatment, age, and overall physical condition. A few popular authors have done a great disservice to people with AIDS, in my opinion, by suggesting that "powers of mind" are the most important factors in healing a physical condition. This con-tributes an added burden—that of feeling like a failure if one's condition worsens. But it's not an either/or situation—either physical or mental factors being primary. We are in the early stages of understanding mind/body interactions, and we will all benefit from studies that can demonstrate what role the mind plays in physical healing.

✏ ✏ ✏

Like many of our caregivers, Penny has come to understand a connection between her work and the emotional deprivation of her childhood, and she has learned that her healing and the healing of her clients are all of a piece. Caring for other people in need, she has found a way to heal her own primary wounds. Her parents' neglect and her divorce have influenced her to assure that no one under her care feels neglected or abandoned if she can help it—and she frequently can. And that fact makes Penny "feel real visible." The expression is the perfect metaphor for her.

> I feel seen when I'm alone in the office and someone calls
> and says, "I'm stuck downtown, I don't have a ride, and
> I'm out of breath," and I can say, "Tell me where you are
> and I'll have a cab there in fifteen minutes." I'm seen when
> I can pick up the phone and make it happen for someone.
> AIDS caregiving has become a big part of my life and
> made me feel more solid and whole. I've gained a lot of sense
> of self doing this work and succeeding at it: beginning with
> clients, one-on-one volunteer work where I was so scared
> I couldn't bear to be around people who were dying. And
> learning that not only could I be around them, but that what
> I got from it was gifts—not the gaping wound that I had
> expected, but gifts!

Note

1. From a study in the *Journal of the American Medical Association*, Dec. 23, 1992.

18
I've Learned How to Lose People I Love

Rickey and I met in high school. We were both queer, but we were in a small Texas town where no one had any context for homosexuality. It was like it didn't happen. So we knew that we were together in something different, and we were very closely bound by that. Rickey and I and a few other nerds got A's and awards in school. Nobody bothered us. The teachers loved us. We were fine.

But I knew I wasn't having the same kind of life that other girls were having—and not just sexually—and I didn't know why, or what the words might be to describe the difference between how I experienced life and how everybody else did.

Ever since then, I've felt myself to be about difference in the world. And my work is about providing for difference, allowing for difference, supporting it, nurturing it.

The world of AIDS caregiving encompasses a populace about as diverse as you can imagine. Many agencies and caregiving institutions struggle to reconcile differences between caregivers and people with AIDS by matching based on permutations of sexual orientation, gender, race, socioeconomic status, ethnicity, and various spiritual paths. Carol Kleinmaier understands the value of such efforts but has no personal need to minimize differences; in fact, she embraces them in her clients and in herself.

Since her high school days, Carol has tried to define what makes her experience of life different from that of other people. She identifies as a "transgendered" person—her primary sexual orientation and gender identity is that of a gay man, and sometimes, as she puts it, "a butch dyke." She is also a member of and educator in San Francisco's SM (sadomasochism) community. And she is one of the nation's most respected support group coordinators, one of the city's most eloquent AIDS spokespersons, and a beloved friend to scores of San Francisco caregivers.

> A lot of what this work is about, in the larger sense, is presence. And my presence speaks for itself. I believe that, and trade on it. I put out as much of my transgender identity as I can among my professional colleagues. I don't do it offensively. I think the key is to speak with enough intelligence and clarity and compassion that they can't help but believe me and listen to me. If I were less articulate, I'd be less credible. I try to express my humanity first, and then add the pieces that are harder to swallow.

> Without an understanding and appreciation of the needs, backgrounds, and unique contributions of diverse groups of caregivers, communication is difficult and misunderstandings are inevitable. Efforts to level our differences or to limit the expression of diverse viewpoints endangers our caregiving just as surely as reducing variety endangers any ecosystem. By ignoring, suppressing or eliminating diversity, we unwittingly stem the flow of creativity, the lifeblood of any AIDS agency and its caregivers.

✎ ✎ ✎

Carol and Rickey married, and in 1981, after graduate school, moved to San Francisco where she taught English literature and composition at the community college level. It only took a few years before Carol knew that she was going to lose Rickey to HIV, or that he would "act out his gay life and leave." That inevitability drew her to Shanti Project in 1983, where she believed she could learn something about loss.

When I volunteered at Shanti, the work was so much more powerful than teaching, and it involved my community—the queer community. I had very good success with clients. After a year or so I knew I could do the work at a much higher level, and I wanted to be a volunteer coordinator. It's all I wanted to do. I was so focused on it that I knew it had to happen.

While I was still a volunteer, I asked to facilitate a group for people with AIDS. I was nervous. There weren't many women doing facilitation ten years ago. But the man who had led the group for years before me said, "Don't worry—your heart is your credential," and I believed him. I led that group for three years. That's where I learned. Since then I've taken all sorts of classes and programs and workshops on leading groups and facilitating communication and healing.

When we interviewed Carol she was coordinating over forty-five different support groups, including ones for caregivers, people of color, women, and HIV-negative men. When a group's facilitator can't make it, Carol fills in. She also leads training sessions for caregivers, and is a frequent speaker at AIDS conferences. And yet, she describes herself as shy, and she used to stutter.

There's an exercise in the training, a listening exercise, which I love to do because I know what a gift it is to be listened to. In our dyad training exercise, one person *just* listens while the other speaks for three to five minutes. Then they switch roles. The luxury of being listened to fully, as well as the difficulty of just listening, become immediately apparent. I have a very old and large pain over not being listened to, and of being afraid to speak because of the stuttering for all those years. It kind of disappeared on its own. I don't know why, but I'm glad it did.

Now in our training sessions, when people listen to me, understand me, and I see that what I say makes a difference to them—it's been very healing for me.

One of the most important provisions that an AIDS agency can offer is in the area of psychosocial and emotional group support—for people with AIDS, for caregivers, for family, lovers, and friends of people with AIDS. The majority of those who avail themselves of such support groups say that they are lifesavers.

The groups that Carol coordinates are primarily nonclinical, nonjudgmental, self-directing, peer support groups. Each uses two facilitators who have had intensive training, and who are often long-term volunteers and sometimes people with HIV themselves. The groups provide a safe environment where peers can discuss HIV issues and express their feelings about what they're experiencing relative to the disease and its challenges.

The first thing I teach in the facilitator training is what makes the space safe, and how you achieve that. The facilitator models and reinforces an atmosphere of respect, nonjudgment, willingness to listen, and empathy. A participant is also assured of freedom from unsolicited advice and from interruption.

Then I structure the training on what safety is in various situations. For instance, integrating new members into a group means protecting the vulnerability of both the new members as well as the existing ones. Facilitators also learn how to stop domineering or judgmental members from intimidating others.

Participants are there both to receive and to give support. Mutuality is understood when you enter the room. Information is shared on all levels, from medical treatments to doctor/patient rela-

tionships, from feelings about loss and death and the struggle to survive to feelings about love and peace and spiritual blossoming.

Groups discuss skills and techniques for managing stress, anger,
depression, and the relentless roller coaster of AIDS uncertainty. In
these places members are free to speak without fear of censorship.
Many of the groups become family in the healthiest sense. Group
membership has become a crucial psychological coping strategy for
many people, particularly for long-term survivors.

But starting a support group isn't easy, and sustaining it is even
harder. Carol's experience as a teacher gave her some basic tools for
the work, and then she went looking for the more specialized intelligence she would need.

A very valuable experience for me when I was learning
about facilitation was working with a group of other adminis-
trators of group programs in San Francisco. We met weekly
to present our models using the group as participants. In this
way we were exposed to ten different support group models,
and many different ways of handling things.

Ultimately, it's a whole process that results in the successful
group programs that Carol oversees, from the agency's in-depth psychosocial assessment of the individual, to placing that individual in
the right group, to having instructed the facilitator how to integrate
new people.

Some groups fail because they are not really peer groups. For
instance, a heterosexual group may dissolve because the women in
the group are of much different backgrounds from the men in the
group, and their agendas are so completely different that there is no
meeting ground. The mistake here is in the constitution of the
group. What works is putting people with similar concerns in the
same room. Carol says, "The desire for connection with peers is so
strong—it's why they come to the group. They want to connect, so
they do."

The initial psychosocial evaluation usually lets Carol know if an individual needs more clinical support than her groups can offer. Occasionally, this is discovered after the individual has joined a group. A person manifesting significant psychopathology, for example, can be a disruptive influence in a group composed of vulnerable, open people. The support group is not designed to provide psychotherapy and will not meet the needs of such a person. When facilitators recognize a person who's obstructing the group's process and who needs more specialized help, they can quickly refer that person to a clinician.

I think it's because they recognize what's working and what feels right in an interaction. They're very well educated in group dynamics and attuned to how individuals affect the group. They're constantly monitoring the room. When something is wrong in the group they're sensitive to it; they know something isn't right even if they can't say why exactly.

＊＊＊

By the time Rickey was diagnosed with HIV in 1991, Carol knew quite a bit about the disease and a lot more about loss, but she still wasn't prepared for his death. She was with him in the last stages of his illness in December 1992.

He had progressive KS in his lungs. He had long since decided that he didn't want to die in a prolonged and painful way, and Peter, his lover, and I both supported that.

Rickey spent three or four days prior to his death talking about how his body was turning to light in different places. And talking about this small spirit whom he called Ariel who perched on his body and was with him. I'd go over after work and lie with him in bed and he would tell me about this wonderful spirit being.

When I wasn't with him, lying with him, listening to him talk about spirits, I was a wreck. A total wreck. Right at the front door I was a wreck. But when I was with him there, it was wonderful. I lay with him and listened, and I believed in his visions. He was making a journey that I was just in awe of. He began to hold off on the morphine drip because he was so into that spiritual journey. He wanted to see more of the spirit and more of the light.

He described launching out of his body with Ariel, and becoming afraid, and coming back. And then they sprang to the edge of the world, and Ariel leaped off and did somersaults, as if to say, "It's okay out here," but Rickey wasn't ready to take the leap with him yet, and so they came back.

He was on very few medications. He was clear, incredibly clear, right up until ten minutes before he died. But then his breathing became labored and then it was clearly painful and not good. At the end, Peter took Rickey's pulse and said, "It's only a matter of seconds." And it was.

During the period of Rickey's dying, Carol was "a total wreck," except when she was with him in that otherworldly space he had begun to inhabit. The words tell us how torn she was about his leaving. There were no mixed feelings, however, about the other world she listened in on through Rickey's narration. She accepted his version of things. She believed his experiences with Ariel had meaning and purpose. She did not jump to categorize them as hallucinatory, or as symptoms or evidence of some sort of strange psychopathology.

I believe it was her allegiance to Rickey that enabled Carol to share his dramatic shift in consciousness. In their long relationship, Carol had been an open and nonjudgmental partner. She was still, and now that openness led her to listen without judgment, but with awe, to Rickey's fear of taking the irreversible leap with Ariel. She believes that something real and even healthy occurred in those shifts that allowed Rickey to encounter Ariel.

Such visitations are not uncommon.[1] The "escort" who accompanies some dying people into the other realm is often a religious figure or a loved one who has gone before. When the environment has been safe for the dying person, I've also observed changes in consciousness that seem to reflect phases of ego dissolution occurring at the end of life. Dismissing such experiences as simply hallucinatory or symptomatic of the disease process may rob us of an invaluable opportunity to learn something about dying. Various Eastern and Western religious traditions and parapsychological studies recognize that in the period just prior to physical death one is more likely to experience these altered states of consciousness. Whatever they represent, such experiences as Rickey's with Ariel may be crucial to the person who is afraid of letting go of life, no matter how awful life has gotten. They helped Carol too, who had been so afraid to let go of her soulmate.

> I came out of it with a very strong image that my job with Rickey was to prop open the door between being alive and being dead, and this door was very heavy metal, thick as a vault. And I was somehow able, through all I've gotten in this work, to stand there and prop open the door and let him go. And that gives me a sense of real power that I can do that.
>
> I think if someone can go so far as to help the person closest to them out of this world, and accept that, and be prepared to act on it, the world doesn't hold a whole lot of fear after that.

◢ ◢ ◢

After Rickey's death, Carol recognized a shift in herself. The worst had happened, and she had survived. "The world can't take anything more significant away from me than Rickey," she told me.

> I know there are people left to lose, and things and capacities I can lose, but I've learned how to lose people I love. But with Rickey's death I also had to address the issue of how to survive in this work in this much pain.

The question, "How can I survive in the midst of so much pain?" is one that every caregiver will eventually ask. Carol has made her life's work answering that question with the help of the hundreds of people with AIDS and all those dedicated AIDS caregivers and group facilitators whom she serves.

> This work is about moving through it whole, finding ways to do that, to come out intact. I think of my support group facilitators who have HIV and how much I love them. We enter into an intense relationship, work together for two years or more, and then I watch them get sick, and they tell me they're leaving, and then they die. After each round of these wonderful people has died, there's always the question of who will be the next ones, and I can name them. And the next question is, can I get through it?
>
> You make a bargain: You'll engage with life knowing that the price for living is loss. If you ever go back on the bargain, that's where burnout and failure take hold, and your work is finished.
>
> After ten years I can't fully engage with everyone, but I do a very good job of taking care of most people, and I think it's because I know I'm capable of living at a very high level emotionally in spite of death and loss, which are givens in this life. I'm able to accept loss as a part of the bargain.

◢ ◢ ◢

Carol says that her sexual ties with the SM community speak to her ability to live "at a very high level emotionally," which is what she believes allows her to live healthily in the world of AIDS. "When I talk about SM, I talk about it in terms of heightened experience and awareness and connection," she says. "I don't talk about pain—it's not necessarily relevant to a broad definition of SM."

Carol says that her participation in SM "play" helps balance her participation in AIDS work, and that it has given her a deeper appreciation for how individual caregivers need to find their own path through this difficult terrain. Though she says "it's not necessarily relevant," I believe that for Carol, SM play may be, in part, a way of mastering pain that one can control—as opposed to the pain of the pandemic that one can't.

> A lot of the same impulses and emotions that are part of my SM play are also part of my work. Both require that I give my full attention. Both require the capacity for intimate connection. Both are creative acts.
>
> It's as if the closer to the edge I get with the work, then the closer to some other edge I have to get to balance emotionally. It has to do with living, with being alive.
>
> I first began to play around the same time I began volunteering. The woman I was playing with was whipping me and I cried. And I recognized that the tears were from a much deeper place than I ordinarily had access to, and I wanted to pursue this path that took me to parts of myself that I wanted to know.
>
> The play became more intense as the years of working in AIDS accumulated and the losses grew and my involvement and energy became more and more devoted to AIDS work. Finally I had to ask myself if I had gotten so far out in terms of loss and grief at work that I was becoming careless about the risks I was taking in play. I thought I might have lost the balance, but I think now it was the intensity of play rising to meet the intensity of work at that time. It told me that what appears to be unacceptably painful can be chosen and survived.

How easy is it to accept Carol's lifestyle? For many folks it's not easy at all. She may challenge us: we may discover that we're not as nonjudgmental as we had thought.

This is a process that prospective caregivers learn about pretty quickly. AIDS caregiving can mean intimate contact with people very different from oneself. Lesbian and gay caregivers may develop close ties with the kind of straight person they might never have related to before. Straight people may learn tolerance in a caregiving relationship from transgendered people, or drag queens, or sex workers. White caregivers with little comparable experience will become students of many cultures. At the same time, volunteer caregivers in the AIDS community must be prepared to see things they have never seen before, things that might initially frighten or anger or intimidate them—and to all these things they are asked to be tolerant and accepting and nonjudgmental. It's asking a lot.

I think that's why many volunteers come to this work. They're willing to stretch, to grow spiritually and emotionally. I think the bottom line is that it is possible to establish connection, humanity to humanity, no matter what the trappings are.

AIDS levels a lot of the differences—a lot is cut away from the beginning. Whatever the differences are, they don't seem very important to me—not when you're talking about loss and death and survival. My friend, Clark Henley, called AIDS "enlightenment at gunpoint." People are knocked out of their superficiality pretty quickly with AIDS.

Note

1. K. Osis and E. Haraldsson, "At the Hour of Our Death," New York, Avon, 1977. A report on deathbed observations in the United States and India with 500 dying patients. Three out of four had such visions.

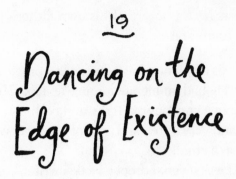

19

Dancing on the Edge of Existence

I used to notice advertisements in the bus that said, "Become a Shanti volunteer," and I thought I'd like to do that but I thought it would be too heavy. I thought people with more skills than I had did that kind of stuff.

But I was losing so many friends, I had to do something. My best friend and I volunteered together at Shanti Project in 1985.

This was the beginning of Alex's commitment to a second full-time job. Weekdays he worked for Pacific Bell; off-work he became a peer counselor with Shanti, a support group facilitator for people with AIDS, spending Saturdays at the Peter Claver Community of Catholic Charities in San Francisco. His attendance record at special AIDS awareness and fund-raising events further demonstrates his devotion to the cause.

Although he had hesitated, insecure about his qualifications, when Alex Martinez came to work with Shanti he already possessed many of the ingredients that would make him an exemplary caregiver, including a kind of sensitivity to another person's pain. From his earliest years he was aware of his own father's pain, and was frequently the brunt of it.

> My father was fifty when I was born. He worked all his life as a waiter. He had immigrated from Mexico, and had two children from a previous marriage, and both had died. He was angry and very bitter, and a lot of his anger was taken out on me as a child.
>
> When I was seven, I dropped a typewriter—it didn't even break—but my father was drunk and to teach me a lesson about the value of things he lit a match and held the flame to my arm and burned me. I was stunned by that. I didn't understand it. As a child I never understood any of his behavior, other than to know it was directed at me.

Alex didn't understand it, but on some level he believed that he must deserve it. He had a miserable childhood, and high school, where he was ridiculed as "the school fag," was little better. He made two attempts at suicide.

> I moved away from home with my very first paycheck. I started living my life, and I really believed I was out of there, so I must be fine. I wasn't. I had been wounded very deeply. In my early twenties I got into bad relationships and I was irresponsible in terms of my health. I did a lot of drugs because they were a great escape.
>
> I used my personality, which, thank God, is outgoing and funny, to compensate, to cover up all that other stuff. I'd do drugs and party and dance all night.

Alex's self-destructive behavior was very likely the continuation of what his father had begun. His father's abuse had caused deep psychological wounds and feelings of worthlessness. Many men and women with similar histories are dragged down by their pasts, succeed at their suicides, or settle for lives of despair. Alex's resourcefulness, intelligence, and good fortune contributed to his survival.

What turned it around for me was this: In 1982 I ended up in the hospital, and I knew I had to change the way I was living. I knew I was desperate for connection, desperate for someone to touch my heart, and I was surrounding myself with people where it would never happen. So I went into therapy. I started. I took that first step.

I had met this guy Rick who had moved to Lake Tahoe and kept inviting me to come visit him there, but I always had made an excuse because I was too busy doing drugs on weekends. The next time he called, I said, "Okay, I'll take the train." I'd never taken a train before. I had never been out of the city. I'm the ultimate city slicker.

It was spring. The train went up into the mountains and the snow was melting so there were rivulets of water everywhere. Rick picked me up in Truckee. That weekend he took me to the top of Heavenly Valley. I had never seen anything like it.

Just as I looked up at the top of the mountain, the setting sun touched the ridge and sent out this flash of orange light. It was the most beautiful, incredible, natural thing I had ever seen. It was as if the light was a laser and reached all the way to where I was standing. It struck me that "You're part of this. You're standing here on this rock by this lake under this sun and you are part of it. You're not some worthless thing—if you're a part of this you must be something." It was as if I had stepped out of myself for a second, and when I popped back in, I wasn't the same person who had walked to that ridge. That moment on the mountain was the purest moment I've ever had.

Alex marks that "peak" moment as the foundation for his caregiving work, because "I learned to love myself." That nature provided a ray of light to commemorate the moment so piercingly, was surely a gift.

According to the psychologist Abraham Maslow, who helped

found both the humanistic and transpersonal approaches to psychology, "peak," or "self-transcendent experiences," are akin to mystical experiences, in which one feels connected to all the universe.

Such experiences may have a profound, even transformative effect. It was so for Alex. Telling him that he was part of something much bigger and more beautiful than his wounded self, it gave him the impetus to begin his healing. It opened an empathic part of him that had been closed off for a dangerously long time. He would find that resource—empathy—invaluable in his caregiving work, as would his clients. Further, he discovered that access to his empathic center allowed him access to other moments of peak experience, and that every such experience moved him further along a healing path.

Alex attributes his healing, which "is a constant process," to finally feeling his pain, really examining it. Therapy has given him one arena for this, the world of AIDS has given him another.

> That's where having been wounded as a child became a
> strength and an asset. I've felt pain and know what it's about.
> I can identify with it when I see another person going through
> the pain of loss, or isolation, or disconnection. For so long I
> thought it made me weak. I used to think that because I was
> a wounded person I was incapable of connecting with anyone.

His AIDS work has taught Alex otherwise. It has provided a place where he can connect in a loving relationship with others who are wounded, and a place where his service to them allows for great personal growth. "I think you can only do the work year after year," he told me, "if you let it transform you." Alex tells this story about his friend Greg, as an example:

> Greg was dying. He was in critical care and he asked to see
> me. He was barely lucid and very weak. I communicated
> with him the best I could, saying how glad I was that he
> wanted me to be there, talking about things we'd done
> together, just talking quietly.

Eventually, I got ready to leave, and I told him I'd be back in the morning. Greg lifted his arm, which was like a bobby pin. With his last bit of energy, he pulled his oxygen mask away from his face and said, "No, no, please don't leave. You give me peace." And then he let go of the mask and it snapped back on his face, and his arm fell.

I caught my breath and told him of course I'd stay. We were in a moment where all I could do was look at him and try to tell him that I loved him through my eyes. As I stared into his eyes I could feel him leaving. I was letting him in as much as I could into my heart, and there was this moment, this encyclopedic moment that passed into me right before he fell into a coma, just before he died. I almost touched what it was like for him. I was as close as I could possibly be. It left me with this openness of heart that I never felt before. It affected me on a cellular level.

When we asked AIDS caregivers, "What was your best care-giving experience—when was it most effective and most fulfill-ing?" the responses were told in stories such as this one of Alex's. Such intimate moments can change us profoundly. A hospital room becomes sacred space, communication becomes communion, an intuitive awareness and deep recognition of the other. Caregiv-ing itself assumes different proportions, "puts you in touch with the ultimate human experience, life and death in all its glory and hor-ror. As the years go by," Alex confides, "I'm actually motivated to continue doing the work in order to make that exploration, that journey."

I asked him if he could enunciate his vision of caregiving, based on his experience.

I think working with AIDS or life-threatening illnesses, we're dealing with edges. What happened to me on the mountain was the edge of our existence. When Greg died he went over the edge of his existence. People who are dying are nearing that edge.

I see people with AIDS struggle to define the edges, to keep control of them. One will decide that when he is finally blind, he'll commit suicide. But then he becomes blind and he says, "I don't want to commit suicide now, but when I can't walk any more, then I'll commit suicide." And then when he can't walk, he says, "I don't want to commit suicide now, but . . . ." The edge is a constant negotiation. I dance around the edge of existence, and it's not such a horrible thing.

- - - -

After several years of doing one-on-one peer counseling, some Shanti volunteers become support group facilitators. Alex is one of these.

We meet at Shanti, and the group varies as people go away to the hospital, and then come back, or sometimes don't come back. John had been in the group for two years when he was hospitalized. He was in a bad way and was going to be moved to another hospital in San Diego to be near his parents, and he asked if the group could meet once on the ward before he left.

I thought it was a great idea because we don't always have the luxury of closure with people. I took it to the group. It had to be a group decision. And there wasn't anybody who said no.

John was attached to pumps and monitors, and had tubes running in and out of him, and he needed a lot of help getting into his chair, but he was lucid and he was very thankful that we were there. He didn't have the energy to engage, but he thanked everybody. There wasn't one of us who wasn't teary-eyed.

It was interesting to me that the two-hour group wasn't entirely about visiting John in the hospital; it was about doing our group. One guy was going blind, another guy had just lost somebody, and we talked about those issues too.

Alex's support group demonstrated its commitment to its entire membership by this unanimous agreement to visit John. That Alex sought the group consensus without interfering in their decision-making process made their decision that much more meaningful. And it made the *group* more meaningful. All the members understood now that the group would be there for them if they were too sick to come to meetings. Their decision declared that no one would be forgotten, abandoned, avoided, not grieved.

The visit to John provided the closure Alex had hoped for the group, and very likely for John, and it did more. It acknowledged the advanced stage of John's disease. Because John was going home to die, it brought the reality of dying up close to every member. And this is an emotionally charged reality that often triggers a deep dialogue—with oneself and with others—about how to live with HIV disease. This is one of the reasons that the support group needs to be a safe place where each individual's reality is respected at each phase of life.

Everyday reality in the world of AIDS is a different reality from that when AIDS is at the periphery of one's experience. AIDS affects everything. Alex occasionally talks to students to try to define that world for them, the AIDS reality as he sees it:

I ask them to imagine for a moment that in their circle of friends 80 percent of them die. Imagine it. Try to. It's an intensely emotional and mind-boggling thing. It can't help but make you question who you are, what it all means, and how you love.

I'm in a relationship now with somebody who's healthy but HIV positive, and I struggle with everything I know and what I've seen doing this AIDS work, to have as much hope as Michael does. I have to hope that he's not going to get sick for years. I have to hope that they'll come up with something for people who are HIV positive.

But it's difficult. Whenever I meet a new person who
is HIV positive, I automatically have all these perceptions
because of my experience, feelings of potential loss, potential
pain. It's hard because I also know that I have to keep my
heart open to it, when the natural reflex is to close up.

We like to believe the adage that experience is the best teacher.
But that's not quite right. Informed, examined experience is the
best teacher. And so Alex struggles. He is a naturally enthusiastic
and energetic man whose optimism might be overridden or contra-
dicted by what he has seen. He struggles against the contradiction,
the negative possibilities, against hopelessness, in order to come to
his clients, and his lover, with an open heart.

As caregivers, we want to think clearly; we want not to judge
our clients; we want to look at each person and his or her symptoms
as unique. These are noble goals, but without our knowing it, our
unexamined expectations may erode our clarity and influence our
thoughts and actions to reflect unnecessary judgments after all.
Alex is aware of this, and sometimes catches himself making
assumptions based on history rather than on the present. He told
me about listening to a client of his talk about opening a flower
shop when he got better, and Alex had thought, "No way. He'll
never make it." He thought it even though he has had many a cautionary lesson in this regard. Martin's was only the first, early in
Alex's caregiving career.

Martin was in his forties when he discovered he had AIDS. He
and Alex spent two years together. When Martin could no longer
walk, he got a motorized cart, and asked Alex to take him to
Marine World. Martin was a big man, 6' 7" tall. They got him into
his cart with some difficulty, and then Martin took off.

It was early, 7 A.M., before the park opened. Marine World
has all these rolling paths and cement waves, and there was
nobody there. I expected that he would motor around slowly
and I'd walk alongside him. But Martin was like a kid in the

motorway at Disneyland. No way could I keep up with him—I mean, he was motorized! He went zipping all over the place. He loved it. And seeing him that way, I didn't see somebody dying any more. I had never seen him so alive.

Alex had some assumptions he hadn't been aware of—he assumed that a man with AIDS in a wheelchair is totally disabled, and that such a person moves slowly, edging toward death. For a moment Alex hadn't been seeing Martin, but his own stereotype of a man in a wheelchair. To do the best we can for those people we care for, a key is to maintain a focus on *this* client and this client's manifestation of HIV rather than to base our expectations solely on what we've imagined, or heard, or been taught, or even on what we've seen.

Each of our clients deserves every opportunity to be the exception to the rule about survival, longevity, and suffering with AIDS. Except in conditions of extreme and destructive denial, the last thing we want to do is contradict, even subtly, the hopeful fight for life that may be necessary for such positive possibilities.

I don't mean to promote a Pollyannish point of view that downplays the physical realities of the disease. Every AIDS caregiver discovers that AIDS is much more than a psychological or spiritual challenge. One of its many lessons, however, is that although we've been taught that seeing is believing, the reality can be quite the opposite. In fact, our beliefs influence and shape what we see as much as any lens might. If we consider all the painful situations that Alex has seen as an AIDS caregiver, it's easy to understand how what he has seen might affect what he believes about a client's chances in a given circumstance. And it's not so hard to imagine how Alex might communicate those beliefs, perhaps unintentionally, to his client, and how that could affect the client's own beliefs and confidence, and by extension, the client's chances of living successfully with AIDS. As a caregiver, Alex has agreed to support his client. As a lover, he has made a similar commitment to Michael.

How can Alex reconcile his anxiety about Michael and "have

as much hope as Michael does"? He'll try not to project his fears. He'll trust that he has the strength and intelligence to take things as they come.

At home, Alex's caregiving experience is sometimes a blessing, sometimes a burden. He has developed great competence and compassion as a caregiver, but he is sometimes plagued by painful images and memories that make family caregiving especially anxiety-provoking. Living with someone with HIV disease means grappling with new occurrences, new information, ups and downs, depression, elation, and more. If Alex allowed his fear of loss to limit his love and intimacy with Michael, he would surely deny himself the full potential of their relationship. So if they get bad news, Alex will ask how serious is this, what can we do to compensate? If they get good news, Alex will celebrate the moment. Such moments of tension and release punctuate their relationship, a relationship they intend to stay and grow with, and live to the fullest for years to come.

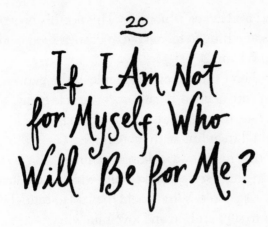

20

If I Am Not for Myself, Who Will Be for Me?

If I am not for myself, who will be for me?
But if I am only for myself, what am I?
And if not now, when?
—Hillel, a Jewish teacher, writing in the first century B.C.

These words of the rabbi and scholar Hillel capture the spirit behind John McGrann's story. He asked the same questions, and found the answers in a ministry among people with AIDS and those who care for people with AIDS. He has come to accept himself, to be "for himself," but to be for others too. John is a Catholic priest. He is HIV positive.

> The people at St. John of God parish know I'm HIV positive, they know I'm gay, they know about my work—they know a lot about me. I told them I was gay in the context of a talk about compassion. I gave them a personal example. I said, "When I told my mother I was gay, her response was, 'If I've ever hurt your feelings, I hope that you'll forgive me.'" To me that's compassion.

Then I told my parishioners, "This is probably going to give you something to talk about at dinner: God made me gay. It's who I am."

Since then I've had several people in the parish confide to me that "my nephew is gay," or "my uncle is gay, and you've helped me see that he's just a human being, and I love him more, and I'll treat him with more respect."

The other night I was talking to a priest who is HIV positive, and it's a secret. I asked him what would happen if he told his people. What could they do to him? The ones who want to support him and love him will.

John sounds sure of himself, and he is—now. But he hasn't always been as comfortable or as public about his sexual orientation as he is today. He grew up the oldest of twelve children on a farm in Washington state. He was barely a teenager when he left home for the seminary, where he tried to bury his sexuality in service to the church. In 1967 he was ordained a priest.

But for all his devotion, John could not deny that vital part of himself. In 1980 he made a trial separation from the priesthood and came to San Francisco. It was a big step. Leaving meant freedom from "so many secrets and so much hypocrisy in the church" around the subject of homosexuality, but it also "meant leaving the people who loved me and were good to me." And it meant leaving security, income, home, and job.

I was very scared and lonely at first. Then I joined a support group—my first—of gay men. There were six or seven of us. My mouth must have been wide open at that first meeting. It was a totally different experience for me to be around gay people. I thought, "God, these are just human beings."

I talked about my feelings and my hopes and my sadness and what was going on for me, and it really felt great! It was through this that I decided to leave the ministry and just take care of myself, get life back inside me, and explore what it meant to be a gay person. I really didn't have a close relationship with anybody, not even God. I had thought I had, but not really.

I bought a florist shop and ran it for a while. But I missed my ministry; I wanted to work with people with AIDS. But I didn't know how I would do that.

John returned to the active ministry, but the church agreed that he would support himself financially. He became the chaplain at Seton Medical Center. He wasn't very happy there, but he met people with AIDS at Seton, and made a commitment to do something to help. To begin, he undertook an informal survey of fourteen different AIDS service organizations in San Francisco, asking them all what they needed most. The answer was consistent: emotional support for AIDS caregivers.

━ ━ ━ ━

At the same time I was doing this survey of AIDS organizations, I had become close to a man named Steve who was dying of AIDS, and I talked to him about what I was finding out, and the ideas I had.

Steve's family was real supportive of him and his lover. It was an inspiration to me. It was at his memorial mass that I shared with people that I wanted to open a place where caregivers could meet. These people were so enthusiastic that they gave me a couple of hundred dollars right then. I made up a couple of pages of names of people who might help or be interested in the project.

I had brought it up before with other people, who said, "You don't know how to run a nonprofit. You don't have a board. Where's your money going to come from? What are you talking about?"

I got Seton Medical Center to fund a brochure that would explain our purpose. That's how Kairos started—from that money and that list of names. I called together some friends to be the first group facilitators.

And so Kairos Support for Caregivers was born in a lovely old Victorian house on a hill overlooking the Castro district in San Francisco. It is a sanctuary for physically and emotionally depleted caregivers—professionals, volunteers, and people who are caring for loved ones. They come together regularly for support groups, celebrations, and personal rejuvenation. It is a house full of love. But it has had its growing pains.

At one point we weren't doing well financially, and I put it to our board of directors—I said, "I've done all the fund-raising up to now. I've got to have some support from you. It's your job. I'm going to leave this meeting and let you folks decide how you're going to raise the money." And I walked out.

And when I left they decided to close Kairos, and not tell me. We went ahead with a fund-raiser, and the board planned to use that money to try to merge Kairos with another agency. I wondered why they were all so interested in how much we had taken in at the end of the fund-raiser!

I was very angry when I found out. My job was at risk. I felt betrayed, disappointed, unsupported, and I couldn't believe that they didn't realize how important our work was— that it's not just a nice thing to be doing, that it's absolutely essential that we support people who are with someone who's dying, that it makes a profound difference.

But I rallied. I didn't give up. I got some people together and said, "This can't happen," and got it going again, with a new board.

I've always figured that if the community needs us we'll continue to have the funds we need, and the caregivers asking for support, and the volunteers.

Kairos is a replenishing station for caregivers, a safe haven, a community in which they find affirmation, recognition, acceptance, and concrete advice about how to handle certain aspects of their caregiving roles. It is also a place where they can temporarily

set aside the role of caregiver and express other aspects of themselves. One thing John knows from his training as a priest is that
any model of caregiving that conceals important personal truths,
that denies self-disclosure, also minimizes the possibility of personal healing, and compromises how much one can effectively do
for another.

As we've seen, the very best caregiving occurs when the giver is
also the receiver. And the biggest single obstacle to the best caregiving is the powerful distinction we are likely to make between *us*
and *them*. *We* are the volunteers, the health care professionals, the
priests, the caregivers, the pros. *They* are our clients and patients;
they are the wounded souls. The distinction may be too hard and
fast, but it is understandable. Caregivers engage in daily confronta-
tions with helplessness and fear. Separating ourselves from our
wounded clients is how we may unconsciously defend against feelings of fear and vulnerability.

The support groups at Kairos allow AIDS caregivers to explore
what frightens them, what hurts in them, where they are vulnerable. They learn that both participants in a caregiving relationship are wounded, and both are healers. This information enables
them to break free of the caregiving model that designates the
caregiver as healthy and the client as the only one in need. In the
process, they often discover that they are too concerned about
being "useful," or that their personal ideas or agendas or desires are
getting in the way of their hearing the person they are caring for.
When John realized this, his one-on-one caregiving style changed
dramatically.

In the past when people came to me and shared their problems, their anxiety, their pain, I'd feel so sorry for them. I'd
think, What shall I tell them? Who should I refer them to?
What book can I recommend? What advice can I give?
How can I fix it so they'll feel better? After a while I realized
people weren't doing what I suggested anyway.
Once in a while, when I had the common sense to shut

up and just listen, the person would say at the end, "You've helped me so much. Thank you for all you've done for me." And I hadn't done anything. I was just there. So I began to get the idea that I didn't have to do anything, and that people didn't want me to fix them, and that I didn't have to take on their pain. I just needed to listen with an open heart that understood and shared what they were feeling.

This is how we help those who come to Kairos. Like Mary, who came to our support group because her son was sick with AIDS. I didn't think she'd come back a second time. She was overwhelmed with sadness and a feeling of helplessness. She believed her son was a victim and there was nothing she could do to make a difference.

But she did come back, and she's really changed. She's been able to talk about her own fear of dying. And she's learned that just being there for her son, just loving him, is enough, is the most precious gift.

✔✔✔

For John, self-acceptance meant coming to terms with his homosexuality, his need for love, his desire that others accept him too, and his HIV status, before he could care deeply for others—before he could even be accepted by others.

I struggled with my sexuality for so long. Sometimes I just cried. Sometimes I was depressed and angry and frustrated. I know a lot of gay people who are so angry that they're gay. "If I wasn't gay," they say, "I wouldn't be dying." "If I wasn't gay, the church would love me." I understand because I went through a long period of not accepting myself and of being ashamed before I came to self-acceptance.

Now that I can better accept myself, I'm valuable to people in a way I never imagined I could be. When people tell me they're lonely, I know what they're talking about because

I've been in touch with that part of myself and accepted it about myself. When they say they're scared, I know what that is. I'm as wounded as they are, and people connect with that.

It is in the evolution of the wounded healer that John faces his own pains before he can effectively enter into the world of another person's pain. He has come to believe that the process of self-awareness requires acknowledging one's own wounds, one's deepest regrets, one's most profound hurts—and then accepting those wounds and regrets. He sees those steps as necessary for people with AIDS and for their caregivers in order to build and maintain a beneficial healing environment.

I agree with John. I think it is *vital* that those of us who care for people with AIDS accept ourselves for who we are deep down. Not perfect. Bruised. Even wounded. And when I say we must accept ourselves, I mean that we must resist any tendency toward self-sabotage, toward any adversarial relationship with ourselves. We must be our own friends, be on our own side.

Self-acceptance allows caregivers to face the challenges of AIDS work with a minimum of self-blame and severe self-doubt. Self-acceptance lets us say "yes" to life. It means I am a friend to myself, I care for myself—I am the same kind of compassionate caregiver to myself that I try to be for my client.

Self-acceptance first, then acceptance of others. That is the climate for healing. The intimate connection one makes in acceptance, whether that be with one's inner self or with another, is the underpinning of the Kairos spirit, and of John's personal spirit. It is also a cornerstone on which the wounded healer builds a caregiving relationship with a wounded partner. This kind of intimacy was new for John. His church had taught him a different way.

My whole training for the ministry was that you were supposed to be an inspiration and an example, and you were supposed to help people, but you didn't get close to them. They weren't supposed to know you or how you really felt.

I held in the truth about who I was. Now I'm able to express it all—be honest about it, laugh about it. Telling the truth about these things, and about my sexuality, and being HIV positive, has been a big healing for me.

It is interesting that John and his colleagues at Kairos have created a context in which some of the deepest feelings about relationships can be expressed. It is as if he has provided himself with a place for making deep connections, for belonging, for loving, for accepting, for admitting his pain, for celebrating his joys.

He also seeks the comfort of other people like himself outside of Kairos. He belongs to a support group whose members are priests.

I've been with this group for three years—it's been in existence for nine or ten. We've become good friends. We get together once a month and talk and pray together, have dinner. A couple of guys in the group are people I could call any time if I needed help.

But my faith and prayer and meditation and feeling connected to God are my real sources of strength. I talk to God. I lie in bed with God. It sounds weird, but at night I let go and thank God, and sometimes I feel God's love and arms about me. I don't know how people survive without some kind of faith.

John's deepening faith in God is mirrored in his deepening faith in himself. His struggle to accept himself—to come to terms with his sexuality *and* with his desire to be a priest, for instance, once seemed irreconcilable. Self-acceptance makes reconciliation possible, and this is the basis for John's ability to create a healing context in which others can accept themselves.

In Part Two, we'll take a closer look at how AIDS caregivers can be wounded in the process of caregiving, and how they can benefit from a holistic approach to self-care.

Part Two

Healing the Wounded Healer

21

Falling Off the Edge

You walk by one room and there's a KS-lesion-covered foot hanging over the end of the bed, and in the next room someone's heaving his guts out, and in the next room you can hear a person wheezing and drowning in her own fluids, and someone else is suffering in some other way. You feel as if you've walked into a Fellini movie.

It's incredible suffering, and loss upon loss upon loss— people losing their jobs, their friends, their identity as a provider, sometimes their minds. It becomes kind of hallucinogenic at moments. It begins to have this depersonalized, surreal quality, and that's when I know I need to pull back and do some self-care and get some distance from it.

—Bharat Lindemood

Most of the people you've met in these chapters work full time as family caregivers, counselors, volunteer coordinators within an AIDS agency, or as health care professionals in a hospital or in private practice. Each knows the intense pressure of trying to meet the needs of people with AIDS with inadequate resources. Each has stood at the edge of his or her capacity to cope. Bharat Lindemood's description of daily life on Ward 5A at San Francisco General Hospital captures some of the horror of the nightmare known as AIDS, and some of the feelings of those who stand on the edge.

You may not be working full time in the midst of the pandemic. You may be taking care of one person close to you. But as you look after that person, visit the hospital, assume new financial responsibilities, manage your job, and cope with your own fears and pain, you too may find yourself wearing down. You may be moody, distracted, depressed, easy to anger, and in private—or public—close to tears. Other people may begin to notice. Someone will ask if anything's wrong. You may want to answer, "Everything's wrong!" but you don't. You may answer, "Everything's fine." But it's not.

Even when patience and equanimity are qualities you've spent nearly a lifetime cultivating, as Jacinta did, you may still not know where your limits are and when you've exceeded them. For Jacinta, realization came when she shoved someone who had cut in front of her as she boarded a bus. Not the kind of behavior you expect from a nun. Some of our other caregivers in these pages have reached similar crisis points, and in getting there "gained a hundred and fifty pounds," "got in a bad car accident," "ended a twenty-year relationship," "started drinking heavily."

Physician Tom Schiller put it bluntly:

> The way I did my work was killing me. I think what makes me good at AIDS medicine is that I get more emotionally involved than most doctors, but it takes so much out of me. Then all this happened with my back. Three herniated disks, back surgery—I was laid up for six months. For three years, since Frank died, my life has not been anywhere near normal. I don't know that I could get back to normal, if I knew what normal was.

Being immersed in the world of AIDS, whether by choice or by necessity, means you let go of "normal." AIDS, unlike cancer, heart disease, and other life-threatening illnesses, can devastate entire friendship networks and communities. Life and work in such extreme situations do not operate under "normal" rules. Assessing ourselves and our reactions to AIDS work based on criteria that pertain to a more normal life or work context, makes all our behaviors at times seem crazy, or at the least, dysfunctional. In this chapter, we'll look at degrees of stress that occur in AIDS caregiving. In the next, we'll offer a multilevel approach to self-care.

- - - -

Full time caregivers live and breathe a form of chronic trauma. Trauma occurs when an individual is exposed to an overwhelming event that results in a feeling of helplessness, or severe anxiety, or grave danger. Chronic trauma is the ongoing existence of such events and feelings. For our caregivers on the front lines of the AIDS wars, chronic trauma comes with the awareness, conscious or not, of severe psychic danger, wherein crucial coping and defense mechanisms are overwhelmed by intense and at times unexpected blows associated with people's suffering, with multiple deaths, and with the achingly painful feelings of grief and loss.

For AIDS caregivers, chronic trauma is frequently compounded by the stresses of organizational problems and dysfunction, by managements whose mission may be less about high-quality caregiving than about funding and career, by the loss of co-workers who can't take any more, by social problems and inequities and diminishing resources.

Chronic trauma is something like permanent white water, like terrible turbulence and no firm ground. It requires that we do something. The alternative is drowning. Psychologists tell us that the failure to address the emotional and psychological impact of trauma forces us to live it unresolved, and trying to avoid trauma's impact by inhibiting or controlling thoughts and feelings actually serves to increase caregiver stress—and the likelihood of gaining weight, turning to drugs or alcohol, having accidents, damaging relationships, becoming ill.

▰ ▰ ▰ ▰

I've been more willing to face my fears, recognize the signs of burnout, and change the ways I do things. If I hadn't, I think I'd have ended up living a totally empty life.

—*John McGrann*

We've promoted the idea in this book that the best caregivers are wounded healers whose relationships with their clients or loved ones serve to lessen the caregivers' own hurts as well as the pain of their caregiving partners. But some people, particularly the more orthodox among the professional ranks, like to think that the best caregivers are *un*wounded healers, somehow above the pain, serving for reasons of altruism, willing to sacrifice personal needs for the client. Among such practitioners, a caregiver who expresses feelings of limitation and vulnerability is regarded as weak or a failure. Among them, caregiver competence is linked with the ability to keep in check personal needs and the emotional responses stirred up by this work. The message is this: Be strong. Swallow your tears. But one can still drown in one's tears.

I believe that emotional remoteness undermines the essential aspect of effective caregiving, which is not simply altruism, but empathy, that circumstance of resonance that our caregivers have spoken of so eloquently in these pages. And empathy connotes emotional closeness, not distance. The inevitable consequences of taking the unwounded healer approach to long-term AIDS caregiving are "psychic numbing," which can lead to "burnout," and "compassion fatigue," which can lead to "traumatic stress syndrome." These conditions occur when our psychological strategies for coping and defense are inadequate, leaving us traumatized by chronic pain or loss or fear. They are by-products of living in a state of constant trauma without a provision for conscientious self-care.

The most universal response to trauma is psychic numbing, a diminished capacity for feeling all kinds of emotions. Apathy, withdrawal, and lethargy are some symptoms, and sometimes memory loss, and confusion about the passage of time. Numbing is closely related to denial. I've heard the words, "It's hard to believe all this is really happening," from caregivers too many times to count.

For caregivers working with people with AIDS, the process of psychic numbing is one way the mind attempts to deal with persistent grief. Especially for those who experience a series of deaths of people they have grown close to, there may not be time to process the tide of emotion that threatens to overwhelm, before the next crisis occurs. Grief becomes not only a backdrop, but a backlog in one's life, and with every new trauma, with every succeeding death, that backlog is stirred up. It's like opening all those graves again. And so we tamp down our feelings, our psychological pain is reduced—at least for a while—and life experience in general narrows.

The end effect of numbing is burnout. Most caregivers know what burnout looks like, but they rarely recognize the slow insidious change from an energetic, committed caregiver to one who is largely indifferent to the needs of people with AIDS, and bereft of the energy necessary for AIDS work. I'm not talking about transient, temporary feelings that we all experience when we have a bad day, or when a situation takes a turn for the worse. The term *burnout* is accurately used only to describe a persistent, chronic condition of physical and emotional exhaustion. The caregiver may demonstrate cynicism toward the one cared for, or may show a dehumanized perception of the client by labeling him or her in a derogatory way or by treating him or her insensitively. Long-term caregivers who have grown progressively numb may evaluate other caregivers as overly emotional or heading for trouble because they don't maintain what the stressed caregiver deems appropriate boundaries. The burned out caregiver may begin offering his or her own psychologically defensive coping style as advice: "Don't get emotionally involved with the people you're caring for!"

But of course, if there's one thing the stories in this book have told, it is that you *will* get emotionally involved with the ones you care for. You must, in order to make your caregiving work for the recipient. You must, in order to heal your own emotional wounds.

Psychic numbing and burnout reduce the caregiver's capacity to feel anything—grief *or* joy. As one becomes more numb, one's client or loved one is perceived as less and less human and more and more a unit of service. You hear him or her referred to as "the CMV in Room 12," or "the user in the waiting room." Caregivers who have come to this can no longer empathize with clients or with other caregivers. They feel progressively disconnected emotionally from what's going on around them, and no matter with what high ideal of altruistic fervor they began their caregiving effort, they find themselves engaged in the antithesis of beneficial caregiving. They have lost the energy for caring and compassionate action. Ultimately burnout will force them to the sidelines.

✐ ✐ ✐

I had a patient who took all his anger out on me. Once he called me a "cunt." A remark like that is hard to let go of. I asked Ron who worked with me and seemed to handle people's misdirected anger better than I could, how he did it. He said, "Sometimes you can't handle it. You have to say 'That's inappropriate,' or 'Quit that.'" That helped me be able to say, "I don't like that," and feel I had the right to say it.

—*Joellen Sheerin, R.N.*

Burnout is different from what we used to call battle fatigue but what I have come to think of as compassion fatigue. It's a condition that shares some symptoms with burnout: depression, anxiety, hypochondria, combativeness, the sensation of being on fast-forward, an inability to concentrate. The difference is that with compassion fatigue, caregivers can still care and are still emotionally involved.

Caregivers heading for burnout begin unconsciously to suppress or wall off more and more of the strong feelings that accompany their work. Those experiencing compassion fatigue are able to monitor this decrease in empathy and feeling and remain emotionally accessible. But they describe greater and greater difficulty in processing their emotions. They are anxiety-ridden or distressed. Fellini-esque images intrude on their days and nights, painful memories flood their world outside the caregiving arena. After too many deaths, too much undigested grief, pain, and sorrow, the caregiver who does not employ numbing as a coping style may well experience the kind of "flooding" that accompanies compassion fatigue. It's important to know that both numbing and flooding are common—we might say "normal"—responses to the savage assault of chronic trauma, and both are evident in many AIDS agencies, in caregiver networks, and among families, friends, and lovers of people with AIDS.

Psychic numbing and compassion fatigue are the results of two very different styles of coping with the same arduous emotional and physical reality—AIDS caregiving of long duration. Neither is chosen consciously by the caregiver. Either may emerge in the course of the work: one style attempts to stave off strong emotion, the other tries to remain open to it, beyond human endurance. In both cases, if self-monitoring and self-care are absent, there's trouble.

Increasing compassion fatigue of long duration may result in traumatic stress syndrome, a more serious mental disorder. Symptoms include intrusive memories, panic and startle reactions, and recurrent nightmares. Some of these same symptoms may occur during compassion fatigue, but more episodically and with less intensity.

✎ ✎ ✎

If someone you know, or you yourself are experiencing burnout, or incipient traumatic stress syndrome, then serious intervention strategies are necessary, such as complete withdrawal from frontline caregiving, or even from AIDS work entirely, and/or professional help. But what if you're not in these extreme states of depletion, but you recognize symptoms of psychic numbing, or you notice some evidence of compassion fatigue? The distinction is an important one in terms of deciding what to do.

If you're experiencing psychic numbing, you need to withdraw from active caregiving for a while, or join a support group, or see a psychotherapist familiar with the stresses of AIDS caregiving. If you don't, then something or someone will cause your withdrawal—an illness, an emotional breakdown, an accident, or someone telling you in plain English to leave.

For those caregivers who think, "I'd love to take a break, but I can't, I'm the only one—" or "it's my livelihood—" or "there's so much to do, they need me so desperately—" keep in mind that dysfunctional caregivers can severely jeopardize their clients' or loved one's care.

We often misattribute the stress we experience to personal problems or inadequacies. Psychic numbing and compassion fatigue are not conditions that have anything to do with ineptitude or irresponsibility. They have everything to do with tragic situations that one may have given one's heart and soul to. In these cases, it is not the caregiver who's "bad," it's the situation. The philosopher Nietzsche once said, "Some situations are so bad that to remain sane is insane." Without adequate psychic and social support, AIDS caregiving can be such a situation.

22

Self-Care for the Whole Person

One of the reasons I'm still here, passionately committed
to living, even with my T-cell count under 100 for over five
years, is my work. I believe God has some work for me to
do, and I've been blessed with the gift of poetry to do it.
If I didn't have it, I wouldn't be here.

—Wayne Corbitt

Caregivers can learn an important lesson from Wayne: because
most people with HIV disease want to live, *a caregiver's principal
role is to support a person with AIDS in his or her struggle to stay
healthy and to survive.* But caregivers who have spent many years
with people dying of AIDS, who have seen too much suffering and
gone to too many funerals, may begin to expect death to be the outcome of HIV disease, and may unintentionally develop a death-
affirming attitude, communicating their expectation in many subtle
and not-so-subtle ways.

What a disservice to people passionately committed to living to
have a caregiver, however well-intentioned, certain they were going
to die! So far, we don't know how much weight to give psychologi-

267

cal factors in the healing process, but it is safe to say they have some effect. Certainly there is growing interest in this subject among researchers in psychoneuroimmunology and practitioners of many forms of alternative healing. On an interpersonal level, this means that what we say or don't say may have an effect on the other. A caregiver must continually check his or her attitude toward a client's or patient's comments about living a long life, or even beating the disease. The will to live, and day-to-day quality of life of people with AIDS are surely affected by the beliefs and attitudes of the people around them. Except in rare cases, supporting another's will to live should not be considered as colluding in false hope; it is assisting in the marshaling of energies necessary to fight for life.

Something else we learn from Wayne and from other people who have been living with HIV for many years is that the struggle against the disease necessitates a commitment to health that is beyond the norm. These men and women work hard to stay alive. They are constantly vigilant in regard to health indicators such as chronic fatigue, loss of appetite, the persistence of cold and flu symptoms, and other signs of ill health or stress overload.

It doesn't make any sense that caregivers be less committed to their own health than to the health of their clients or patients. And yet, caregivers sometimes entertain the peculiar notion that self-depleting sacrifice, particularly the sacrifice of one's own health, is all right if it can be construed to be in the service of someone with AIDS. A caregiver's self-depleting sacrifice, maybe especially of his or her health, is not all right and doesn't serve anybody. In fact, caregivers must be especially vigilant because some of the stressors that afflict them are frequently insidiously subtle. They creep up on us disguised as a bad day or an irritability, but they can be more than that, and once entrenched become more and more difficult to shake.

There's a debate among caregivers and caregiver supervisors about whether a careful, considered focus on one's own well-being isn't really the equivalent of selfishness; about whether asking another caregiver to lend a hand doesn't demonstrate flagging commitment on your part; about whether taking a workshop in self-care or seeking counseling isn't an admission of weakness or lack of ability. It's not. It doesn't. It's only smart.

The alternative to burnout, compassion fatigue, and the symptoms of chronic trauma that often confront AIDS caregivers is self-care. You may not have thought much about self-care before you got involved in AIDS work. All that has changed. Now it becomes a priority.

— — —

What I try to do in my life is to embrace all of creation—
which will include the nightmares.

—*Micaela Salort*

In presenting a multilevel approach to self-care, I've borrowed a useful analogy from psychologist Larry LeShan, who has specialized in working with cancer patients, and who likens their situation to a nightmare. Three circumstances apply: one, terrible things are happening to you; two, you are helpless—there seems to be nothing you can do to change what's happening; three, what's happening goes on and on, seemingly endlessly.

Ongoing experience with AIDS, for the one who has it and for the one who cares for someone with it, can come to feel like an absolute nightmare. If all three conditions above exist—the terrible things, the inability to stop them, the no-end-in-sight—then it is a nightmare with a nightmare's special ego-weakening and emotionally and physically exhausting effects.

If all three circumstances apply and we care about our clients deeply, we become painfully aware of how much they need, how enormous their personal struggle. We may even conclude how hopeless it all seems. And when an AIDS caregiver comes to the conclusion that the situation is hopeless, he or she has breached that most important caregiver principle: to support the person with AIDS in his or her effort to strive for health (emotionally, spiritually, and as much as possible, physically) and to survive.

◢ ◢ ◢ ◢

How do we caregivers keep a life-affirmative outlook for ourselves and our clients? How do we withstand the assaults, and even
turn the tide toward life? We intervene in the original equation,
the siege formulation of bombardment, powerlessness, and forever.
We address each of these components with a different kind of
intervention.

Level I: Changing the Channel

The first level of intervention focuses on the bombardment aspect
of the nightmare: you're living a tidal wave of people with AIDS.
Or the one you love most in the world is dying from it. Or the people you're trying so earnestly to help turn their anger and frustration
at you, as if *you* are part of their problem. You begin to measure time
in funerals; your world darkens. Bharat Lindemood described the
experience this way:

> Driving to work, what stands out for me is the gray concrete
> of everything, pollution, darkness. I don't see the light any
> more. I remember taking a message off the office answering
> machine from a patient on another ward. The voice said,
> "Hullo, I'm in Room 5-C-12. I need to talk to someone,"
> and I was suddenly so overwhelmed by the amount of suffer-
> ing. I wished I could push that voice back into the box.

The caregiver who is struggling against darkness needs to redis-
cover some of life's light. He or she needs to change the channel, by
which we mean the most basic, even obvious type of individual
intervention, where the caregiver purposefully turns away, if only
temporarily, from the horrific images and dark thoughts, to some
positive alternative. For instance, you would do one of these:

1. *Establish a regular exercise regime*—one you enjoy—
at least three times a week. Lisa Capaldini has taken up sculling.
"It's completely useless. It does no good other than to get me out

with the seals and the birds, and it's great exercise. When you scull, the ideal is to get into a rhythm that becomes almost a meditation. It's a very mindful thing, which is a nice model for being with my patients."

2.   Or *adopt stress reduction techniques* that quiet the mind and calm the body, like meditation or yoga—also three times a week or more. Eric Poche does tai chi: "Tai chi is important for me. I can't sit in lotus position. It's just not me. Tai chi is both graceful and centering, and it's vital."

3.   Make a commitment to *weave revitalizing activities into your life*—like massage, walks in nature, quiet time. For Richard Jackson, it's time with his dogs, who provide "100 percent unconditional love." For Danny Castelow, it's time at the end of the day: "My apartment has an incredible view, and every night I sit and look at the city skyline and take in my day. Sometimes when I come home late and I'm really tired, I don't feel like doing it, but I do. It's a kind of closure at the end of the day."

4.   *Build in time-outs and/or time-offs* so that you can vary the intensity of your work. Even if you're the sole caregiver for someone you're close to, you can take a break of several hours, and sometimes of several days. Remember that almost every caregiver in this book has mentioned how crucial it is to have time to himself or herself that has nothing to do with AIDS. Alex Martinez makes an annual excursion to Hawaii. "I never went to Hawaii until AIDS. It's wonderful. I'm away from phones, from problems, from my beeper, my group. As much as I love it, I need to get away from it."

* * * *

Changing the channel involves choosing activities that take you out of the caregiving role and as much as possible, away from anything that might remind you of AIDS. This minimum self-care approach may include movies, hobbies, gardening, sports, music, hot baths, dog walks, cooking, and/or potboiler fiction.

Level II: Getting Outside Support

While changing the channel is vitally important to your efforts to transform the nightmarish quality of the situation, it is not sufficient in containing the ongoing stresses of AIDS caregiving. Level I intervention offers necessary but temporary relief only. When Alex comes back from Hawaii and Lisa puts the scull away, the siege resumes.

Level II addresses siege condition number two: you feel helpless to make a difference. Your efforts on behalf of your client with AIDS feel like drops in the ocean. Even your own attempts at self-care don't seem to make a difference. It's vital to remember that you're part of a caring team of people. If you're a sole caregiver, reach out to AIDS agencies or a network of friends for help.

I have long been struck by the fact that more Vietnam vets have died from suicide after the war than were killed during the war. This is the potential toll of traumatic stress syndrome, perhaps no less so for AIDS caregivers on the front lines who suffer compassion fatigue or endure chronic trauma for years and receive little or inadequate support.

Outside support may occur in a variety of contexts, which we'll look at below. What all these support systems have in common is that they provide psychological resources *while you continue your caregiving work*. Your feeling that you can't cope with this by yourself is accurate. You can't. You don't have to. Don't even try. Instead, do one or more of the following:

1. Tell your stories to a friend or colleague who is familiar with AIDS work.

2. Seek professional help from a counselor or psychotherapist, preferably one who is familiar with the stresses of AIDS caregiving.

3. Participate in caregiver training.

4. Join a support group for AIDS caregivers.

All these approaches are ways to share what you're going through. Sharing your pain with another person lessens the burden you carry back into the caregiving arena. Sharing your experiences helps validate them. Sharing your feelings and thoughts evokes responses from others that may help you—insights into ways to handle certain situations that you may not have considered.

Telling Your Stories

What is good for the person with AIDS is frequently also good for the caregiver. We have seen the importance of bearing witness for the person with AIDS, of acknowledging his or her suffering and experience with the disease. The caregiver's need for witnessing is equally important, whether it occurs in a one-on-one sharing of stories with a friend or loved one, or with a psychotherapist, or in a supportive group of other caregivers.

But this is not common intelligence. Many caregivers report that no one wants to hear their stories or acknowledge their suffering. Many feel less worthy of that attention than their clients. But why should that be? Why should the presence or absence of a molecular-sized virus determine which person is listened to, which one commiserated with?

So when co-workers, or a loved one, or an agency asks, "What can I do for you?" think about what Micaela Salort says: "If you're going to be in my life, you're going to have to deal with the intensity. I'm not going to talk to you about trivia." Ask the person who wants to help to agree on a good time in an emotionally safe place for you to tell him or her your stories. And if no one asks, caregivers can initiate such opportunities to tell their tales, preferably off-site, outside the workplace.

We need our powerful emotions to find expression, but there's frequently an ambivalence about experiencing and expressing strong feelings—as if we may open a Pandora's box in doing so. Penny Chernow confesses to being "one of those people who avoids dealing with grief as much as possible, because when it comes out, it comes out." But to avoid the danger of not letting it out at all, Penny has found a safe way to express and to attend to this dimension of her emotional life. "When I cry, they are tears from my whole life. When someone dies, it's not the loss of one person, it's about all the losses of my life. So sometimes I go to a very sad movie on purpose because I want to let it all out. It feels good."

It's natural to fear being swamped, maybe drowned by painful emotions. But suppressing the feelings our caregiving work stirs in us doesn't eliminate them by any means; it only puts off the inevitable face-off to a time when our defenses are low.

One-on-One Professional Help

Most of the caregivers in this book engage in, or have engaged in some form of one-on-one psychotherapy or counseling. In many urban areas, especially in large cities, free or low-cost therapy for AIDS caregivers is fairly accessible. Mary Corwin has two therapists. "I'm only slightly screwed up," she says. "They're both women. One is just for me and the other is for Sinead and me. With one I dump whatever feelings overwhelm me that I can't figure out what to do with. I don't always get answers, but it's like naming a fear. Once it's named, it's not as ferocious."

Many caregivers will benefit from counseling or psychotherapy, especially if the therapist understands the extraordinary demands of AIDS caregiving. Jacinta's counselor is a Jesuit priest who has been involved in AIDS volunteer work. "I see him every couple of months, just to touch base," she told me. "He encourages me to talk about my AIDS work at home in my religious community. I used to think I couldn't do that."

The caregiver's relationship with the counselor or therapist, like other significant relationships, takes time to develop, and evolves over more time. Caregivers frequently think that what they *don't* have is time to invest in a self-centered psychotherapeutic process. And then they are amazed at how much time it can take to recover when they have been struck down from the pressures of unrelieved caregiving work. Then an hour a week seems a small price to pay.

One-on-one support is crucial for caregivers who have HIV or AIDS and who wonder if they will have any friends or loved ones left to care for them at the end of their lives, or for caregivers with AIDS who wonder whether suicide will be an option at the end of their lives. One-on-one support is also crucial for caregivers who are HIV negative and suffer from survivor guilt, a kind of sympathetic distress that seems only fair in light of the clients' suffering. This feeling of guilty regret can escalate to the feeling that it's "only fair" that the caregiver join his or her departed friends, loved ones, or clients. Survivor guilt is unlikely to be relieved by the individual strategies for self-care discussed in Level I.

Caregivers who work with a psychotherapist in order to enhance their own healing frequently are able to recover their sense of purpose and the almost spiritual sense of mission that brings many caregivers to AIDS work. Recalling the original intention and commitment to the work, and exploring why that has dimmed, often stimulates a compelling set of reflections. For example, the caregiver may see how a particular work setting has kept him or her from fulfilling earlier, idealized intentions, or how emotional exhaustion or overwork has limited his or her ability to respond constructively to human problems.

Training

There is no substitute for on-the-job training in AIDS caregiving, but most of the caregivers you've met here would agree that more formal training specific to AIDS caregiving is also vital. Shanti Project has, for twenty years, provided a solid multiday training program for volunteers at the beginning of their work, and made further training opportunities available to volunteers on an ongoing basis.

In addition to learning about taking care of people with AIDS, caregivers are also educated in the normal reactions to chronic trauma. They are warned of the dangers of repeatedly stifling strong emotions. They hear the credo of the wounded healer: that acknowledging and understanding one's personal wounds, instead of denying them, is key to effectively adapting to work stress and will assist one in sustaining a genuinely compassionate attitude toward one's clients and oneself.

Support Groups

Support groups, safe havens, opportunities outside the workplace for trauma debriefing, for sharing one's suffering and insights and wisdom, have become a permanent feature of the AIDS landscape. Larry Hjort explains why:

> If you're dealing with a life-threatening illness you have a lot of issues that are very personal and very difficult, and if you don't talk about them, you end up holding them in and they're not resolved and they become intolerable.
>
> The group process is really important to help you acknowledge your feelings and get feedback from other people. It allows for bonding with others, and provides a commonality of feelings that you don't get watching people talk about AIDS on Phil Donahue.

The support group is where we share feelings about loss and death and relationships and the struggle to survive. We tell how we manage stress, express our anger, and handle depression and uncertainty, the handmaidens of the AIDS pandemic. We bolster our social support systems with these groups; we learn about our communities' resources.

Such groups allow us to see what's common to us all. From this we gain perspective on the sources of our stress, like inadequate resources, insufficient funding, dysfunctional organizations, or the simple numerical reality—too many people to serve, and not enough of us to do the work.

Wisdom Circles, a New Model for Support

Wisdom Circles is a meeting format being pioneered in the San Francisco area for the purpose of mutual support. It shares some aspects with more traditional support groups: participants sit in a circle and speak about difficult personal issues; it allows for protected time and space to reflect on major life events and transitions. It differs in that it does not employ a facilitator, and it ritualizes the group process in order to maximize the safety, confidentiality, and trust that are necessary for self-disclosure.

Each wisdom circle begins and ends with a shared experience of the group's choosing. This may be a silent meditation, each person lighting a candle, a prayer, an invocation, a song, or any other symbolic action the participants agree on.

A ceremonial object designates the speaker: when a group member is in possession of the stone or sacred book or "talking stick," the other members bear witness, listening from their hearts, without judgment. The emphasis in a wisdom circle is on gaining insights from one another's direct experiences as revealed in each speaker's story. Therefore, there are no interruptions, no advice is offered, nor any effort made to "fix" the situation about which the speaker is speaking. For the speaker's part, he or she communicates from the heart as truthfully as possible. When the speaker is through, he or she passes the ceremonial object to the next member who wants to speak.

Many of the very demanding aspects of caregiving work around such issues as death, suffering, love, or compassion can be introduced through ritual in a wisdom circle. By lighting a candle to represent loss, for example, or filling a goblet full of water to represent love, a speaker provides a tangible focus for the group's attention and his or her own story. We seem to be able to access a deeper part of ourselves through ritual than by ordinary discourse. In the caregiving wisdom circles I've participated in, we have also used guided imagery exercises for that purpose. Rituals and such exercises are not common to traditional support groups.

I believe that both support groups and wisdom circles are necessary for us to share the deep challenges we face in this work, as well as the major insights about love and service that are also part of the world of AIDS caregiving. Survival as an AIDS caregiver is a collaborative process. Nobody survives without help. I can't overemphasize the importance of joining a support group or starting a wisdom circle (see Appendix). If there isn't one in your area for caregivers, start one, or ask an AIDS agency to start it.

Level III: Seeing the Bigger Picture

That third circumstance that exists when the caregiver's world has become a nightmare is that there appears to be no end to the dream that is all too real. The sense of neverendingness is relieved by entering larger domains of human experience in which AIDS plays a smaller part, or no part at all. Level III interventions are appropriate when Level I activities like physical exercise, meditation, time off, and entertainment—all the usual and necessary health maintenance and stress reduction techniques aren't enough—*and* you also see a therapist and attend your support group faithfully— and you're still icily numb or constantly fighting back tears. Level III is designed to reorient the caregiver so that he or she can see the bigger picture, life's larger reality. At Level III, we readjust our sights. This is a two-part process that asks us to designate an important life goal separate from our caregiving work; and to search for a way to connect with our spiritual selves.

Setting a Life Goal

Some AIDS caregivers are notorious for having little outside life, for having their primary lives and deepest, most meaningful involvements within the caregiving world. Others believe that their families and friends cannot offer them the intimate connection, attention, and respect that their clients provide. Sometimes they try to function as caregivers with their own families and loved ones, and may feel hurt when their efforts are rejected or not appreciated. Soon, all their efforts, time, and energy are turned toward AIDS caregiving and away from other personal needs.

Caregivers *must* have a life outside of AIDS caregiving or risk becoming overly dependent upon, even "addicted" to their work. Caregivers must check in with themselves frequently, even during the hardest times, to ask, Where am I going with my life? What do I want from life *in addition* to the gratification I get from AIDS caregiving? A life goal is based on values we hold dear and that excite us to learn, create, and grow. A life goal motivates us to proactivity. Our engagement with it signifies that something healthy is occurring that is unlike our caregiving work, even though our caregiving may also be realized as life-affirming. The life goal enlivens us. We take pleasure in its fulfillment. For Eric Poche, that thing that enlivens is his woodcarving work. Cecilia Worth's creative life is expressed through her photography and writing. Richard Jackson gains the deep pleasure I'm talking about by working to perfect his karate. Alex Martinez sees his life goal as co-creating a relationship of soulmates with his partner.

We all know it's important to set life goals and to design steps to achieve them, but how many of us have taken the time to do either? And yet, working toward a meaningful life goal changes the feeling of life, sometimes substantially. With a life goal, we aren't merely reacting to life's circumstances. We become architects of our own lives; we no longer feel like pawns in the AIDS game. We have expanded the directions in which we can move.

A commitment to writing, music, or art, or any worthy goal, can enrich your life and expand its meaning. A life goal such as raising your children, or keeping a spiritual path, or pursuing ecological issues, requires that you grow as a person. Pursuits that provide new insights and that heal old wounds will allow you to bring more wisdom and perspective to your work as a caregiver.

━ ━ ━

It's not a matter of serving the client with AIDS or serving oneself. The more self-aware and resilient I am and the more I develop my capacity to learn and grow, the greater my capacity will be to serve others. And the opposite is true: the more compromised my physical resources, emotional resilience, and mental stability, the less effective I become in serving others.

The Spiritual Connection

I'm a true believer in God, not in organized religion, but in my own personal sense of the divine. I trust a higher power. I pray every day, I grew up with that, and I have conversations with God: "What the hell is all this about?" or "What am I going to do now?"—stuff like that.

—*Eric Shifler*

What I have heard, listening to the caregivers' stories in these pages, is their deepening realization of what it means to be human. This is a part of seeing the bigger picture. For me, this includes the ability to experience and express deep feeling, and a heightened awareness of the sacred in everyday life—by which I mean a sense that life, however tragic, deserves our reverence, respect, and gratitude.

Like Eric, I don't equate spirituality with organized religion, although I know one may find nourishment for his or her spiritual hunger there. And it's my observation that personal growth is frequently stunted when spirituality is seen as a remote, or otherworldly phenomenon. When you work in the world of AIDS, the work and the experience are immediate and couldn't be more down-to-earth. It is spiritual work because it evokes in us a sense of communion with something larger than ourselves.

George Simmons, who claims to have become less spiritual as a result of his AIDS work, provides a good example of the kind of spirituality I mean:

AIDS caregiving has changed what I appreciate about life. Quality of light, for instance. I know that sounds crazy, but last New Year's Eve I was at a party at a house by the ocean, and the light in the room was so pretty, and the sound of the surf in the background just filled me with happiness. I was sober, by the way. That's my definition of a spiritual moment.

Millions of lives worldwide are being shattered by AIDS. But it's also true that within the tragedy, and perhaps because of it, profound insights are occurring that are leading many people to a deepening vision, purpose, and faith in life. Finding insufficient answers outside for the tragedy of AIDS, many of us are compelled to look to our deeper selves, and sometimes to eternity for answers.

It is within the greater reality that we enter in pursuit of our life goals, and within the spiritual dimension, that we are able to confront the never ending aspect of the nightmare we call the AIDS pandemic. In fact, from the point of view of some caregivers, the physical suffering their clients endure is a nightmare that only ends at their death, but other caregivers, and many you have met in these pages, demonstrate that there is psychological and spiritual healing to be found in the darkness. Our caregivers may not achieve a permanent end to the nightmare, but they find moments of profound respite for themselves. Daniel Warner, who wrote the foreword to this book shortly before he died, said that for him AIDS stood for Accelerated Inner Discovery of Self. I think Danny was right; AIDS is certainly a cruel teacher; yet it is one from which we may learn much about kindness, love, and the eternal.

A Time to Stop

Many people who become long-term caregivers or who work as staff for any of hundreds of AIDS agencies throughout the country began by caring for a beloved friend or family member, and afterward were motivated to do more. Working at the front lines of this awful assault for five or eight or ten years takes a toll on even the most resilient and resourceful caregiver. At some point it may be necessary to stop. Gary Shepard spoke poignantly about that decision.

In a real way, one's leaving the work is inherent in doing it, just as death is an inevitable part of life. When I stopped volunteering, I did so because I needed to pay attention to myself. I believe that service can never be only an outgoing function. There always comes a time when repair work is needed.

Having said that, I don't know of any ardent caregiver who doesn't fear stopping on some level. I know I did. I wasn't the same person I had been before I started the work. Without the work, I wasn't sure I'd know who I was any more. Who or what would contain all that grief? Who would really understand what I had been doing? All of the people who really knew, who were in the room with me, are dead.

I don't have answers for these questions, but I know they're important to the issues of caregiving. To stop is to experience aloneness and isolation and the mounting fear of beginning again.

I always come back to the notion that this work is never about what you do, but about who you are, or perhaps, who you are becoming. The answer to stopping may lie somewhere in there—that you go on becoming, finding kindred spirits, healing as you go. But caregivers need to be given permission to stop. Maybe there should be a training for stopping, like there is for beginning.

Maybe Gary is right. Too often we expect always to be strong, efficient, and in control. When problems arise, instead of reaching out for help, we may assume the blame (by thinking that we are weak, inefficient, out of control) and we may try to hide the problem and the presumed cause, from others. Soon we are awash in anxiety.

To avoid this trap, it's necessary that we care more for ourselves, for the emotional, psychological, social, spiritual, and physical aspects of ourselves. This is holistic healing we're engaged in; therefore, each aspect deserves attention and expression.

✐ ✐ ✐

Our own grief for those who die, our fear of pain and loss, the need to face our own mortality and to continue our own healing and growth throughout our whole life—all these contribute to the necessity for clear and continuous self-examinations in any of the ways we have suggested here: through wisdom circles, support groups, psychotherapy, artistic commitment, spiritual disciplines, personal introspection, or other individual means for giving voice and vision to the further reaches of our human nature.

The Future of AIDS Caregiving

I think it's clear by now that acknowledgment and support are vital for those people who work and sometimes live in the vortex of trauma and loss that are part of the AIDS pandemic. As they grow in wisdom and experience, AIDS caregivers and the staff members of AIDS organizations that support them are fast becoming a treasure that we cannot afford to squander. We must protect our committed caregivers from burnout, compassion fatigue, and the effects of chronic trauma at the same time we continue to draw more volunteers and professionals with organizational and caregiving skills into the fold.

The future of AIDS caregiving will need more organizations like Kairos Support for Caregivers in San Francisco, a place dedicated to providing comfort and solidarity for those folks on the front lines. There are severe limitations in relying primarily on individual solutions for alleviating the stresses of AIDS caregiving. Quick-fix stress management is not the answer. Addressing the root causes of caregiver distress is.

A caregiver-sensitive environment can promote nurturing personal and workplace relationships and help caregivers avoid excessive isolation. AIDS organizations of the future will need to acknowledge the toll of AIDS work by providing mental health days, adequate bereavement and vacation leave, and occasional job rotation off the front lines. They may employ the wisdom circle for enhancing communication, emotional expression, and problem solving, and initiate job sharing, team-building, flexible benefit packages, and opportunities for paid caregivers to exchange a percentage of their salaries for extended time off.

✸ ✸ ✸

One important distinction stands out for me with regard to the future of AIDS caregiving: the emphasis of the whole movement is continuing to shift from care for people dying from AIDS to care for people living with the disease. Many of us continue to hope—and we must hope—that the future will ultimately make AIDS caregiving obsolete, at the same time preparing ourselves for the possibility that AIDS will be with us for the rest of our lives.

All the great worldly accomplishments that were deemed impossible—the end of smallpox, the scaling of Mt. Everest, breaking the four-minute mile, putting a person on the moon—became possible because someone or many people believed they could be done. Positive belief, vision, and determination always precede and accompany accomplishing the impossible. I think it's crucial for all of us to hold as a precondition the mind-set that AIDS is curable. I think we'll find the cure only when enough of us believe we can, and want it to happen, and act on that—not instead of financial resources, research, and political action, but as the very foundation for success in these areas.

✸ ✸ ✸

I don't know any caregiver anywhere who would not agree that AIDS caregiving changes your life. You get to see, close up, how agonizing life can be, how fickle, how random, how precious, how sacred. You learn when you act in service to another person, how your life and that other person's life can at times become illumined and ennobled. Service becomes our mirror, that place where we meet each other as reflections of a single, caring consciousness, where we don't try to conceal our pain or avoid it, but share it as an impetus to healing and renewal. In the words of an old Hasidic proverb, "Before we can *be* together, we must learn to *grieve* together."

Appendix
Wisdom Circle Constants

These constants are the guidelines for conducting a wisdom circle:

Honor the circle as sacred space and time by opening and closing it with an appropriate gesture or ritual that creates a shared sensory experience—for example, lighting a candle and remembering someone, a moment of silence, a meditation, or listening to a musical selection.

Create a collective center of attention on one or more of the following: envisioning our future, healing our wounds, going within to learn more about ourselves, making decisions and planning actions that sustain and enrich life for ourselves and others.

Ask to be informed by the wisdom of our predecessors, of all those living today, and by the needs of those yet to join us.

Express gratitude in silence or vocally by turn, giving thanks for the opportunity to be of service to people in need, and for the teachings of this work.

Listen from the heart and serve as compassionate witness to the other people in the circle.

Speak from the heart and from direct experience.

Create a container for full participation so that everyone who wishes to speak may be heard. A "talking stick," or "talking stone," or any other symbolic object may be passed around to signify the person speaking.

Make room for silence to enter—for reflection, for meditation, for feelings to surface as the circle proceeds.

Rotate leadership with the ultimate goal of having a leaderless circle.

Glossary

AIDS: Acquired immunodeficiency syndrome.

ARC: This abbreviation stands for AIDS-related complex, a collection of conditions associated with HIV infection. ARC is a nebulous term that was common at the beginning of the pandemic but is not used now.

Apnea: A temporary cessation of breathing.

AZT (azidothymidine): An FDA-approved drug that suppresses replication of all stages of HIV. Adverse side effects may include anemia, muscle wasting and fatigue, headaches, depression, and nausea.

CMV retinitis: A virus that affects the retina in some people with AIDS, that may result in loss of vision or blindness.

Coccus: A suffix that indicates a spherical bacterium.

Cryptococcosis: A severe fungal infection that frequently causes meningitis (an infection of the membrane of the brain and spinal cord) in people with HIV infection. Common symptoms include vision problems, seizures, fevers, and headaches.

Dialysis: A mechanical process used in the elimination of impurities from the blood during kidney failure.

Epidemic: A serious, contagious disease spreading rapidly among many individuals in a community at the same time.

Giardia (giardiasis): An intestinal infection by a parasitic protozoan that may cause prolonged pain and diarrhea.

Herpes Zoster: A condition often called shingles, caused by the same virus that causes chicken pox. Symptoms include skin sores similar to those of chicken pox that begin as red spots and become water-filled blisters.

HIV: Human immunodeficiency virus that is responsible for AIDS.

HIV+: After HIV enters the body, antibodies to HIV usually appear in the blood. This is known as seroconversion. A blood test indicates either no antibodies (HIV negative), or the presence of antibodies (HIV positive, or HIV+).

IV: Refers to injecting, by needle, replacement fluids or drugs directly into veins.

KS (Kaposi's sarcoma): A kind of cancer of the small blood vessels that affects 20 percent of people with AIDS. Symptoms are purplish lesions or nodules anywhere on the skin, and sometimes on lymph nodes and internal organs. It is the second most common disease after PCP that may indicate an AIDS diagnosis.

Neuropathy: An illness involving the nerves. Most frequent symptoms are painful feet and legs. Other symptoms include weakness and/or tingling in a muscle.

Palliative care: Intervention strategies aimed at controlling a patient's pain and keeping him or her as pain-free, comfortable, and alert as possible.

Pandemic: An epidemic over a large region affecting many communities or even an entire nation or nations.

PCP (Pneumocystis carinii pneumonia): An infection of the lungs caused by the pneumocystis carinii bacterium. The most frequent serious opportunistic infection in people with HIV disease. Symptoms include shortness of breath, fever, and coughing with sputum.

Periodontitis: An inflammation of the tissue surrounding the teeth—for example, the gums.

PML (progressive multifocal leukoencephalopathy): A viral infection deep in the brain found in individuals with severely weakened immune systems, including some people with HIV infection.

Pneumothorax: The presence of air or gas in a pleural cavity, especially as a result of perforation or rupture of the lung tissue.

Septicemia: A systemic disease caused by the presence of pathogenic microorganisms and their toxic products in the blood.

Seropositive: A term used to designate people infected with HIV when they have been diagnosed by a blood test that detects antibodies to the virus.

SM (sadomasochism): As defined by practitioners, the conscious, safe, and consensual use of psychological and/or physical dominance and submission in erotic fantasy play.

Toxoplasmosis: An opportunistic infection passed by contact with feces or infected cats, or ingestion of raw or undercooked meat. It most frequently causes an inflammation of the brain (focal encephalitis). Symptoms include personality changes, confusion, disorientation, headaches, fever, chills, seizures, tremors, shakiness, motor changes, blindness, coma.

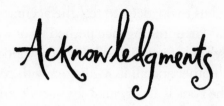

Acknowledgments

Many books are as good as the stories people share. We are first and foremost indebted to the courageous men and women who continue to care for people with AIDS and their loved ones in the midst of a modern day, multinational plague. Special thanks to those caregivers who willingly opened their hearts and allowed us to bear witness to their truths.

Putting together a book is an enormous endeavor. Brief acknowledgments don't do justice to the truth, that a book's personality reflects the personality and passion of every participant. First, let me thank those who worked directly on the project:

Cindy Spring is my primary partner on all aspects of the book's creation. I could easily write ten pages of tribute to her. Cindy's conceptual contributions and impeccable sense of organization are what an author hopes to get from a skilled editor. What has made our partnership significantly different, however, is her passionate concern for the concepts and values we present. This book is about love and service and loss and pain and care and trust. It's also about listening, speaking, and acting from the heart. Cindy's dedication to the deeper meanings of these words has been a consistent inspiration. She urged us to dig deep to test the accuracy of our ideas. Her integrity and keen intelligence pushed us onward in desired directions. Cindy's belief in the possibility of a world in which people relate to each other and all living beings with compassion and respect is what the book is about, what she's about, and what is central to our lives. Best of all, she's my wife.

Doris Ober's skill as a writer has made our subjects come alive. Doris took a great deal of conceptual material and made sense of it, integrating my voice with the unique voices of our caregivers telling the emotionally demanding stories that are the heart of the book. She championed certain wording and slashed the beloved redundancies. Her professionalism and commitment to the work is what every author hopes for in a collaborator.

Bharat Lindemood read the first draft of the manuscript and made many helpful suggestions and incisive comments. The book has benefited considerably from his wise counsel. I feel fortunate to have such an aware and penetrating reader, and blessed to count him as my friend.

Lana Angel has been a model associate from start to finish, transcribing the emotionally charged interviews with our caregivers, courteously fending off intrusions during the writing, arranging my complex speaking schedule, and helping us with intelligence and good cheer whenever we needed her.

Sylvia Garfield, my mother, read the penultimate draft of the book in her chosen role as CGO (Chief Grammar Officer). Mom's careful proofreading unearthed a number of errors and oversights and demonstrated that she is still, at the age of eighty, an astute, valuable, and much-loved member of our team.

━ ━ ━

Lynn Luckow, president and CEO of Jossey-Bass Publishers, approached me directly with the idea for this book. I have known

Lynn for almost twenty years as a friend, and on various projects, as a valued colleague. His courage in introducing books about AIDS to the Jossey-Bass list reflects his unflagging support of people with HIV disease and those who care for them. From beginning to end, Lynn and his colleagues made me feel like family rather than commercial property. It is a thrill to see him emerge as one of the bright lights of American publishing.

Alan Rinzler, our editor, combines the savvy of a publishing insider with the heart of a caregiver, a perfect combination for this book. His intelligent advocacy and enthusiasm for the project showed his colleagues at Jossey-Bass that, in a very personal way, this was their book too.

David Landay is a wise, compassionate soul whose commitment to AIDS issues is legendary on both coasts. He is a networker supreme whose friendship and advice I value a great deal. A number of conversations with David about issues central to AIDS caregiving made all the difference in the world.

Daniel Warner wrote the foreword to the book shortly before he died in June 1993. A teacher until the very end, he showed us that if caregivers really pay attention, they will learn more about life, love, and service from people with AIDS than from anyone else.

Carol Kleinmaier is a kindred spirit in our commitment to bring the highest quality training, support, and leadership excellence to AIDS caregivers. In weekly conversations during the writing of this book, we explored the farther reaches of human caring and compassionate community in an effort to extend current thinking about caregiving. Carol has been the intelligent adviser and nonjudgmental listener that every caregiver would like to know but seldom expects to find.

Micaela Salort has been, like Carol, one of my closest colleagues over the last several years, during which time the three of us have talked endlessly about supporting people with AIDS and their caregivers. Mica has been an important member of my own support team throughout the writing of this book.

✌ ✌ ✌

We are deeply indebted to all our interviewees, each of whom showed us the heart of AIDS caregiving. Among AIDS caregivers today, there is so much of deep importance that people think and feel, but have not yet spoken out about in communities around the world. This creates a special need for our exemplars and their peers everywhere to be the voice for the dispersed and largely unheard caregiving community. If we listen, we will hear them say, "Something very important is happening out here, something basic to the way people relate best to one another, something that makes it imperative that we try to understand love and caregiving in a time of AIDS."

About the Author

Charles Garfield founded and served as board chair and executive director of Shanti Project, one of the first and most inspiring AIDS agencies in America. While a faculty member at the Cancer Research Institute at the University of California Medical School in San Francisco, he originated the innovative approach to peer support later known as the Shanti model. For his work with Shanti and with many other organizations replicating the Project's approach, he was named National Activist of the Year, one of America's highest awards for voluntary contributions to public service.

Garfield was a computer scientist on the Apollo Eleven Project that sent the first men to the moon. Afterward, he launched an ongoing study of high-achieving individuals, teams, and organizations, which inspired his widely respected peak performance trilogy. *Peak Performers*, Garfield's 1986 best-seller, was translated into eight languages and is one of the most influential books on superior achievement. *Second to None: The Productive Power of Putting People First* appeared in 1992 and was one of the few books chosen twice as a main selection by the Executive Program, one of our nation's most prestigious executive book clubs. *Peak Performance*, published in 1984, earned Garfield an invitation by the United States Olympic Committee to deliver the keynote presentation at the esteemed Elite Coaches Symposium, addressing the head coaches of our Olympic sports.

Garfield is a clinical professor in the department of psychiatry at the University of California Medical School in San Francisco and a fellow of the American Psychological Association. His vision of caregiving excellence and of the farther reaches of individual and organizational performance brings him into frequent contact with individuals involved in AIDS caregiving and in the complex issues of health care leadership and reform.

The Charles Garfield Group
3756 Grand Avenue, Suite 405
Oakland, CA 94610
Telephone: (510) 272–9500
Fax: (510) 658–7946

About the Writers

Cindy Spring is director of Syntropy Audio, a nationally recognized producer of nonfiction audio programs. She has adapted the works of numerous well-known authors into the audio format in such diverse fields as health, psychology, business, and self-help. With Charles Garfield, she coauthored the program *AIDS Caregiving: Lessons for the Second Decade*, and has served as structural editor and adviser on his last three books. She is also the cofounder of Wisdom Circles, an organization dedicated to the creation of compassionate community through meeting in circles.

Doris Ober is a writer and personal editor for many Bay Area authors. She worked with Randy Shilts on his last two books, *And the Band Played On: Politics, People, and the AIDS Epidemic*, and *Conduct Unbecoming: Gays and Lesbians in the U.S. Military*. Other recently published books on which she has collaborated are Winnie Smith's memoir, *American Daughter Gone to War: On the Front Lines with an Army Nurse in Vietnam*; and the biography, *Covarrubias* by Adriana Williams.

Index

132–133; self-healing and, 104–105, 106, 270–283
Public speaking, 127–128

Q

Quality of life issues, 107–108, 168–169, 179–182, 225; taking excursions, 197–198
Queer community, 229
Questions: asking patient history, 177–178; perfunctory, 134

R

Racism, 38–39, 55
Raoul (client), 168–169
Rationality: and psychosocial support, 51–52; and sense to the patient, 109–110
Reality: the AIDS world, 245–246; and appearance, 90–91, 246–247; of the bigger picture, 278–283; comparing perceptions of, 133; dealing with, 206–209; major changes in, 216; rejecting another's, 113; reorienting caregivers to, 278–283
Reciprocity in caregiving, 57–58
Records, keeping, 110
Recovery from addiction, 203–208; caregiving and, 209–211
Recovery of caregivers, 274–275
Reinforcement, positive, 218
Rejection: of gay offspring, 17, 181
Relationships. See Caregiving relationships; Intimate relationships
Relationships: periodic adjustment of, 70, 75, 76
Respect: caregiver/patient, 165, 210; doctor/nurse, 113–114; doctor/patient, 74–75, 109; the right to, 41; self, 28–29

Restaurants, going to, 197–198
Reverse discrimination, 222
Richard (Capaldini's patient), 114–115
Richard (Salort's patient), 60
Richard (Sheerin's patient), 133
Rickey (Kleinmaier's friend), 227, 228–229, 232–234
Rilke, Rainer Maria, xiii, 152, 153 n1
Rituals, Wisdom Circle, 276–278
Robbie (client), 118–120
Robert (patient), 105–106
Roger (Garfield's patient), 1–2
Roger (Schiller's patient), 181–182
Role reversals, 9, 50–51
Roles: being deeper than, 161; defining caregiver, 71

S

Sadness, surviving with, 172–174
Sadomasochism (SM) community, 228, 235–236
Safe environments, groups as, 230
Safe sex videos, 222
St. Louis Effort for AIDS, 127–128
Sally (client), 100
Salort, Micaela, 53–66, 146, 273
Sanctuary for caregivers, 251–254
San Francisco, 276; as a city of ghosts, 171; employment in, 206
San Francisco General Hospital, 21–22, 128; AIDS tidal wave at, 139; inpatient Ward 5A, 9, 32, 41, 59, 65, 142–143, 203, 206; outpatient Ward, 85
Saving the world, impossibility of, 162–163, 164
Schiller, Dr. Tom, 75, 175–187, 260
Schweitzer, Albert, 175
Scott (Castelow's client), 36
Scott (Sheerin's patient), 135–136
Screening volunteers, 224
Secrets: need to tell, 23, 159

Sports, 271
Spring, Cindy. *See* About the Writers, 297
Stalling treatment, 46
Statistics, AIDS orphans, 223
Stereotypes, 40, 178, 228, 246–247
Steve (patient), 104–105
Stigma of AIDS, 5, 89–90; internalizing, 150
Stories, 10; letting out, 16–17, 19–20, 30, 209; telling caregiver, 273–274; truth in, 124–125; Wisdom Circle, 277
Straight doctors, 178
Stress, caregiver, 7, 84, 259–260; perspective on sources of, 276; reduction techniques, 271; symptoms of, 260
Strong, being, 262
Stuttering, 169, 229–230
Substance abuse. *See* Drug users and addicts
Suffering and awareness, 56, 149, 159. *See also* Pain; "Wounded Healers"
Suicide, 107, 172, 272
Support systems: for AIDS caregivers, 251–254, 272–278; gay, 96–97, 205–206, 250–251; loss of patient, 7; for women and children, 96–97, 219–220. *See also* Groups, support
Surreality, 259
Surrender: by patient to professionals, 50, 130–131, 175–176; of caregiver's personal feelings, 53, 57
Survival: believing in, 11; of caregivers, 172–174, 277–278; collaborative process of, 86–88, 277–278; denial and, 209; physical and spiritual, 50; with so much pain, 234–235; to tell the story, 16, 30; unexpected, 35
Survivors: living with the disease, 34–35, 225; of lost friends, 24–25, 86, 126, 172–174

Suspicion: between caregivers and drug users, 90, 91, 207; between patients and doctors, 176
Sympathy dependent on origin of AIDS, 89–90
Symptoms: burnout, 263–264; living on without, 225; of psychic numbing, 262–265; talking about, 30, 109–110; traumatic stress syndrome, 265; unpredictability of AIDS, 5, 35, 196–197, 206

T

Teacher, client as, 9, 50–51
Teaching tales, 10
Ted (patient), 29
Teenage drug abusers, 201, 202
Telling: caregiver stories, 273–274; how you feel to the doctor, 134, 177–178; how you got AIDS, 89–90; positive feelings, 218; secrets, 23, 159; that the patient is gay, 185–186; that you are gay, 17–20, 178; that you have AIDS or HIV+, 98, 150, 206, 214; the truth, 124–125, 181–182; your children, 214. *See also* Advocacy; Stories; Words
Terminal care, 106–107, 177, 288; hospice, 60, 133, 191–192, 199–200
Terminal reality of AIDS, 10–11
Terror and anger, 84–85
Tests, having, 21
Therapists, mental health, 125, 129, 232, 274–275
Thomas, Lewis, 113
Time: motherhood and limited, 219; remaining for the patient, 107
Time management: and emotional support, 49–51, 110–111, 274–275, 283; for yourself, 271
Tolerance and hostility, 19